51

DAYS

NO EXCUSES

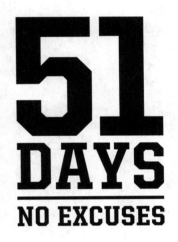

51 DAYS

NO EXCUSES

RICH GASPARI

DUNHAM
books

Author/Publisher Note: This book proposes dietary recommendations for the reader to follow. However, before starting this or any other diet or exercise regimen, you should consult your physician. Consuming raw or undercooked eggs may increase your risk of foodborne illness, especially if you have a medical condition.

ISBN 978-1-939447-13-5 (Trade Paperback)
ISBN 978-1-939447-14-2 (E-book)

Printed in the United States of America

This book is dedicated to my father Stefano Gaspari, a man who came to the USA from a war-torn Italy to better not only his life, but the lives of his children. He taught me that with hard work, determination, and drive that you can be successful in life. He was a loving father and my mentor and I am truly grateful to have had him as my father. I always believe he is looking down on me and is proud of my accomplishments.

CONTENTS

INTRODUCTION

WALKING THE WALK

I hadn't competed in a bodybuilding competition for nearly two decades. I was still highly involved in the sport through my nutritional supplement company, Gaspari Nutrition, attending competitions, and sponsoring professional athletes, but my body wasn't where I wanted it to be.

I wasn't in bad shape, but with my work being done from behind a desk and loads of corporate travel, I felt soft. But what was bugging me even more was that I felt a little hypocritical. Here I was—the CEO of a company that emphasizes fitness and maximizing one's physicality— and I wasn't practicing what I preached.

If I was going to challenge my customers and fans to believe that mediocrity was not acceptable and to reach for their best, then I knew I needed to throw down the same challenge for myself.

Now everyone knows a 48-year-old man can't compete. Right? Some of my best friends let me know it. Of course that wasn't the first time I'd heard, "You can't do it." In truth, I didn't have any real plans to compete again, but I did feel a burning desire to work out like I was going to be in the Mr. Olympia contest. I wanted to get myself into the best shape of my life—not only for my age, but for any age. And one thing you should know about me: I am a very competitive person. Failure isn't an option.

I started on Memorial Day. Fifty-one days later my body fat was down to two percent. Take a look at the cover photograph again and tell me I couldn't do it.

This book is the story of my 51-day journey. But it's not just about me. It's about you. And I'm here to tell you that you can achieve your ultimate body by following the same program.

I don't care if your goal is to be a bodybuilder or just get in better shape—you are going to get leaner, stronger, ripped, and bigger in the right places.

I don't care if other programs haven't worked for you—this combination of diet and workout regimen is going to give you results that blow past anything you've experienced in the past.

I don't care if you don't have all the right equipment, feel too small, think you are past your prime, or whatever other negativity is nagging at you—you are going to look and feel great.

You are going to work out a muscle group every day and you are going to eat seven meals every day—with less fat, more protein, complex carbohydrates, and supplements to fill in the nutritional gaps that you can't get in your food.

There's nothing magical about 51 days. I've heard it takes 40 days to start a new habit, so I believe the extra 11 days will make sure what I am teaching here really takes hold.

Don't miss what I just said. I haven't stopped at 51 days. Now that I've got my ultimate body back I don't have any intention of letting it go anywhere. Because this isn't a quick-fix program. This is a lifestyle.

Are you ready? The good news is I'll be your workout partner every day. I will be in your face letting you know in no uncertain terms that failure isn't an option.

Just a few words of wisdom: don't take this training program lightly; it is hardcore and if you follow it as it's laid out and give the routine 100% intensity, you will undoubtedly build muscle and improve your overall conditioning. The good news is that the secret to more muscle is pretty simple: train heavy and with intensity.

Fuel your exhausted muscles with the right nutrients and enough calories to sustain muscle growth. If you're not eating enough, guess what, you don't have enough raw materials to build your body!

Try to sleep approximately eight hours each night—if you're sleep deprived, your body isn't going to heal and grow after these workouts I have for you. Do it!

Stay the course. If you don't feel like training, realize that you are the only person who can hold you back. Stop the excuses and turn what you think will be a lagging workout, into your greatest workout yet!

Are you ready to get started? Are you ready to walk the walk with me? Let's do this!

—Rich Gaspari

THE DAILY WORKOUT

My overall approach has changed drastically from my years as a professional bodybuilder in my 20s and early 30s. When I was a bodybuilder, I was mostly concerned with gaining mass on my physique and building up for a contest. Back then, I trained on a six-day split. During the off-season, it would be three days on and one day off.

As a contest approached, say 8-to-10 weeks out, then I trained 6 consecutive days. My training during this time would be a double split, where I'd train once in the morning and once at night. I always trained to failure (repeating an exercise to the point of momentary muscular failure), using very, very heavy weights with low repetitions.

Now that I'm in my 40s, my training has changed. I still love training and do it five days a week, but I only train once a day for about an hour to an hour and fifteen minutes. I now train to maintain what I have and to avoid injuries with moderately heavy weight and higher repetitions.

What weight should you work out with? Muscles don't know weight—muscles know and respond to failure. I would suggest you start with a comfortable weight that challenges your limits, but allows you to exercise safely. But the lighter you go the more reps you need to do to reach failure, that point when your muscle says, "no more."

THE DAILY DIET

I hadn't seriously dieted in more than 15 years, and honestly I like the fact that I can eat what I want and stay in fairly good shape. That's a plus. I have good genetics and don't gain body fat easily. But getting in shape like I was when I competed is another story!

The first thing I needed to do was to make sure I ate enough throughout the day, so I would get all the proper nutrients to stay in an anabolic state. And by eating seven times a day like I used to, my metabolism sped up to burn fat and increase my lean muscle mass. I also felt it would be a true testament to my products to use them for my transformation. Myofusion, SuperPump, Sizeon, Anavite, and BCAA6000 are the main products I took for my transformation.

I also know my body responds well to higher carbohydrates that are more complex, so I stay away from white flour and white sugars and eat more of an even distribution of proteins-to-carbs with the essential fats from fish oils, almonds, and natural peanut butter. My protein sources are grilled chicken, lean red meats, egg whites, white fish, and Myofusion, with my complex carbs coming from sweet potatoes, brown rice, oatmeal, and occasional whole-wheat pasta. I get my fibrous carbs from broccoli, asparagus, and green salads. I also eat some fruits: bananas, apples, and one cup of natural apple juice (a half cup each for the two shakes I drink every day).

Stick with these nutrition guidelines and do your best to stay within the guidelines of the eating plan—this will ensure that you're fueling your exhausted muscles and neurological system with the necessary nutrients for ongoing muscle growth and consistent progress throughout your training.

Before we begin Day 1, review the following points:

1. GET A JOURNAL AND START WRITING DOWN EVERYTHING YOU EAT.
You can download free apps for your smartphone if that works better for you. The important thing is to hold yourself accountable.

2. YOU WILL EAT SEVEN MEALS EVERY DAY–and you will include protein with every meal.

3. PREPARE, PREPARE, PREPARE! Eating seven times a day will require that you plan ahead for your grocery shopping and daily meals.

4. YOUR FOOD RATIO CONSUMPTION WILL BE: 45% complex carbohy-drates (fruits and vegetables); 40% lean proteins (my favorite is buffalo meat); and 15% healthy fats that are full of omega-6, such as olive oil, nuts, etc.

5. CUT OUT SUGARS AND GLUTENS FROM YOUR DIET–only eat complex carbohydrates.

6. EAT WHAT YOU LOVE. I will show you what foods to eat, but you can come up with your own recipes. Be creative! If you have some great recipes that work on the program—please send them to me so I can share them with others.

7. MAKE GOOD FOOD CHOICES WHEN EATING OUT. For you to achieve your ultimate body, you can't be scarfing donuts with your coffee in the morning or running out for a burger with fries for lunch. You will learn how to eat smart while on the go.

8. CONSIDER NUTRITIONAL SUPPLEMENTATION. I believe you will need some supplements to get enough protein—and I want you to focus on probiotics and antioxidants. Remember, you get what you pay for—avoid discount brands.

DAY 1 START WHERE YOU ARE

Do you have some extra fat around your waist you didn't have a few years ago? Are you already discouraged because you are doing this on your own and haven't found a training partner? Are you feeling tired before you even get to the gym? Do you feel like you are stuck in a rut in life and are having a hard time getting started? Are you mad that you can't get definition in your lower legs? Or your abs? Or build muscle mass in your chest?

Good. I'm glad you know you are in a big fight and that this isn't going to be easy. The old adage is true. Nothing worthwhile comes easy. But when you achieve your ultimate body, it is going to feel even better. You will know what you fought through.

If you are a little mad, frustrated, disgusted, or whatever you are feeling right now, that's fine with me, because those kinds of emotions are what we all need to make a commitment to change. If I hadn't been a little pissed at myself, guess what? You already know the answer. I wouldn't have accomplished what I did over the course of 51 days. If I had been happy and content I would have stayed on a comfortable course, not pushed myself to the max.

I don't care what shape you are in right now. I care about where you are going. I am a firm believer in looking forward. Achieving the ultimate body—or any other kind of success in life—is a journey based on setting a goal and then having the discipline to work toward it. It's not where you are today that matters. It's having a goal that matters.

When I first decided I wanted to be a bodybuilder, I was a skinny fourteen-year-old kid. I had just been released from the hospital after a three week stay for a bad case of mononucleosis. I don't think I weighed 100 pounds. But I saw pictures of bodybuilders in some muscle magazines a friend's dad had saved in his basement and I knew that's what I wanted to look like; what I wanted to accomplish. That vision of what could be became my goal

If I had focused on what I wasn't and what I didn't have, I would have quit before I started. I had great parents, but as struggling immigrants from Italy, their primary concern was that there was enough food on the table, not helping me accomplish anything in sports. That wasn't the world we came from. In fact, my dad tried to discourage me from body-building. He would tell me, "If you want big muscles, come work with me laying bricks."

My first gym was a corner in the basement of our small house. I found a bench, a bar, and a few weights someone down the street wanted to get rid of. That was it. But it was all I needed to change my life. Why? Because my current situation wasn't nearly as important as what I wanted to become.

My point to you is simple. I don't care if you are broke, too small, too heavy, lack encouragement from others, or have any other obstacles in your way—I've been there and faced each and every one of those limitations. You can still do it. All you need is a goal.

If a goal is a vision of what we want to be, then what I want you to do right now is find a picture that epitomizes what you want to look like 51 days from now. If you don't have some bodybuilding or fitness magazines laying around your place, head for the store and buy one that has a picture of someone with your ideal body. Tear it out and tape it somewhere you will see it often. Now there's no way you can forget you have a goal. You might put it on your bathroom mirror where you will see what your body is today and what it is going to be. That's a great way to monitor your progress.

Just remember, I don't care where you are now. I care where you are going. And when you get your mind and body marching forward rather than stuck on what you have or don't have now, you are already on your way to success.

You can get your ultimate body. How do I know? Because I did it.

DAY 1:
THE DAILY WORKOUT

Each day you will find two different workouts, the Hard Gainer and the Muscle Builder. You decide which one fits you better. A Hard Gainer is someone who has a hard time gaining weight through exercise. If that is you, please follow the Hard Gainer routine each day. Everyone else please follow the Muscle Building routines.

THE MUSCLE BUILDER: CHEST & ABS
(Take 45 seconds - 1 minute rest between each set)
Incline dumbbell press – 4 sets of 8-10 reps
Incline dumbbell flys – 4 sets of 8-10 reps
Decline cable flys – 4 sets of 8-10 reps
Superset: Dumbbell flat bench, Pec Dec – 4 sets of 8-10 reps
Crunches – 4 sets of 25-30 reps
Leg raises – 4 sets of 25-30 reps

CARDIO
20-30 minutes interval cardio on treadmill

HARDGAINER WORKOUT: CHEST/BACK/BICEPS/TRICEPS/CORE
Modified Compound Superset #1 – *Take 45 seconds rest before moving on to the 2nd exercise*
Incline Dumbbell Press: 3 sets of 4-6 reps (45 Sec Rest)
Barbell Bent Over Row: 3 sets of 4-6 reps (1 min rest)
Modified Compound Superset #2 – *Take 45 seconds rest before moving on to the 2nd exercise*
Flat Dumbbell Bench Press: 3 sets of 6-8 reps (45 Sec Rest)
Chin-Ups: 3 sets of 6-8 reps (Strap on weight if you can)(1 min rest)
Note: If you cannot perform the Chin-up, either have someone spot you by using your legs off their hands for leverage or have them spot-push you up by the waist.
Superset #3 – *No rest between exercises*
Barbell Curls: 3 sets of 8-10 reps (No Rest)
Close Grip Dumbbell Bench Press (Triceps): 3 sets of 8-10 reps (1 min rest)

Superset #4 – *No rest between exercises*
Dumbbell Hammer Curls: 3 sets of 10-12 reps [No Rest]
Triceps Pushdowns: 3 sets of 10-12 reps [1 min rest]
Superset #5 – *No rest between exercises*
Plank: 2 sets of 1 Minute Static Contraction [No Rest]
Bicycle Maneuver: 2 sets of 30 reps [1 min rest]

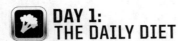

DAY 1:
THE DAILY DIET

This workout was what I did during my 51 day trans-
formation, and the protein and carbohydrate portions is
what is recommended for a man. Females following this
program please cut down the protein and carb portions by
half and use discretion.

MEAL 1: Myofusion Shake: 2 scoops Myofusion, 1/2 cup egg whites, 2/3 cup instant oatmeal, 1 tablespoon natural peanut butter or almond butter, 1/2 cup apple juice, 1/2 cup water and ice.

MEAL 2: Myofusion Protein Pancakes: 1 scoop Myofusion, 1 cup egg whites, 1 cup oatmeal, 1/4 cup chopped walnuts, 1 sliced banana. Mix all together and cook on low heat on a non-stick pan using cooking spray. Optional: add sugar-free syrup.

MEAL 3: Same as Meal 1.

MEAL 4: 8 ounces grilled chicken mixed with 1 cup brown rice, 1 tablespoon olive oil or salad dressing with 1 cup veggies.

MEAL 5: Same as meal 1.

MEAL 6: 8 ounces lean ground beef, 1 cup gluten-free pasta, 4-6 ounces low sodium natural tomato sauce with 1 tablespoon grated cheese [optional].

MEAL 7 [optional]: Same as Meal 1.

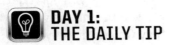

DAY 1:
THE DAILY TIP

The greatest hurdle you will face is convincing yourself that
what you want is possible.

DAY 2 THE NECESSARY NUTRITION

When I decided to transform my body in 51 days, one of the first changes I had to make was to what and how I was eating. I hadn't dieted in years—and by dieting I mean measuring every single gram of food I put in my mouth and eating every meal exactly on time, seven times a day. I had to make sure I ate enough throughout the day so I would get all of the nutrients my body needed and stay in an anabolic state. Also, by eating seven times each day, my metabolism would speed up—burning fat and increasing my lean muscle mass.

Feeding your body quality food five to seven times a day isn't easy. It takes planning, preparation, and often sacrifice. Most people aren't willing to put that kind of effort into their eating. They miss meals, they let too much time elapse between meals, and they don't eat the right things. Guess what? A box of fried chicken nuggets is not the same as a grilled chicken breast. A bag of chips or French fries is not the same as a baked potato or a bowl of rice.

To be sure you always have the food your muscles need to recover and grow, you have to plan ahead and you may need to bring your food with you in a cooler to work or school or wherever you spend your day so you don't get caught without it. In the old days, when someone was so poor they couldn't afford food, they would say they didn't know where their next meal was coming from.

Thankfully, we live in a land of plenty so that's

rarely a concern. But as a bodybuilder, you always need to ask it anyway, you need to know where your next meal is coming from. If you don't eat right you will short-circuit this training program. In particular you always need to have enough protein at every meal. Without protein, your muscles lack the raw building blocks necessary to grow.

What's the difference between this type of attention to diet and what the average Jack or Jill in the gym does? Do you really need to ask? You can always spot the ones that push harder with both their training and their nutrition, because they look awesome. Anyone that tries to down-play the importance of proper nutrition in the big picture of fitness is only fooling him or herself.

It's not easy to make sure you're always stocked up on all the meats, starches, vegetables, and supplements you need. It sure isn't easy to keep meals cooked and packed ahead of time for the whole day when you eat every two to three hours. It's not convenient to always make sure you have the right amounts of the right foods at the right times, every single day. But if it were easy, everybody would have fantastic physiques.

You need to ask yourself this question: just how badly do you want the physique you dream of? Just a little bit? Maybe you'd like to look awesome, your very best, but it wouldn't be a big deal if you never got it. If that's how you feel, you're not ready and perhaps you never will be. But I don't think that's who you are.

You want to be bigger and stronger so badly you can taste it. You close your eyes and you can't stop picturing yourself with so much thick, striated muscle that people will hardly recognize you. You dream about what it's like to own that type of physique, and you are determined to make that dream a reality.

You know it's going to take a ton of hard work and it won't happen overnight. But you're in this for the long haul and you will never quit. You will challenge yourself to train with greater intensity, be totally precise with your nutrition and supplementation, and always be sure your body gets adequate rest between each and every ferocious workout. You don't need someone yelling in your ear to motivate you, because that voice is already inside your head.

Is this you I'm talking about now? Are you ready to push harder every day to reach your goals? If you are, you have come to the right place. Keep reading. You've got a lot of growing to do!

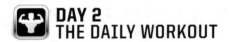 **DAY 2
THE DAILY WORKOUT**

THE MUSCLE BUILDER: BACK & CALVES
[Take 45 seconds - 1 minute rest between each set]
Deadlifts – 4 sets of 8-10 reps
Wide grip chins – 4 sets of 8-10 reps [free form or with chin assist machine]
Superset: Close grip pulldowns, Wide grip cable pullovers – 4 sets of 8-10 reps
Superset: Cable low rows, T-bar rows – 4 sets of 8-10 reps
Superset: Two arm dumbbell rows, machine rows – 4 sets of 8-10 reps
Standing Calf raises – 5 sets of 15 reps
Seated calf raises – 5 sets of 15 reps
Cardio: 20-30 minutes interval cardio on treadmill.

HARDGAINER WORKOUT: THIGHS/HAMSTRINGS/DELTS/CALVES/LOWER ABS
Superset #1
Wide Stance Squats: 3 sets of 4-6 reps [45 Seconds Rest]
Stiff Legged Barbell Deadlifts: 3 sets of 4-6 reps [1 min rest]
> *Note: Utilize the "Full Body Tension Technique": This is when you stay in proper anatomical form and maintain that posture by keeping all of your major muscles contracted before & throughout the movements – This will keep you safe, while allowing you to use maximum intensity.*

Giant Set #2 – *3 exercises performed back-to-back without rest*
Leg Press: 3 sets of 6-8 reps [No Rest]
Leg Extensions: 3 sets of 10-12 reps [No Rest]
Lying Leg Curls: 3 sets of 10-12 reps [1 min rest]
Giant Set #3
Upright Barbell Row: 3 sets of 8-10 reps [No Rest]
Lateral Raises: 3 sets of 8-10 reps [No Rest]
Descending Set #4 – *Drop the weight as you move from set–to-set*
Standing Calf Raises (Gastrocs) - 3 Descending Sets – Decrease weight as you descend, if necessary:

• 1st set of 12-15 reps (15 sec rest)
• 2nd set of 12-15 reps (15 sec rest)
• 3rd set of 12-15 reps (1 min rest & repeat 2 more times)

Superset #5

Bent Over Lateral Dumbbell Raises: 3 sets of 10-12 reps (No Rest)

Seated Calf Raises (Soleus): 3 sets of 10-12 reps (1 min rest)

Hanging Leg Raises: 3 sets of 15-20 reps (1 min rest)

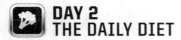 **DAY 2**
THE DAILY DIET

MEAL 1: Myofusion Shake: 2 scoops Myofusion, 1/2 cup egg whites, 1/2 cup instant oatmeal, 1 tablespoon natural peanut butter or almond butter, 1/2 cup apple juice, 1/2 cup water and ice.

MEAL 2: Myofusion Protein Pancakes: 1 scoop Myofusion, 1 cup egg whites, 1 cup oatmeal, 1/4 cup chopped walnuts, 1 sliced banana. Mix all together and cook on low heat on a non-stick pan using cooking spray. Optional: add sugar-free syrup.

MEAL 3: Same as Meal 1. (Or lessen oatmeal to 1/4 cup.)

MEAL 4: 8 ounces of lean steak, 1 sweet potato, 1 cup asparagus.

MEAL 5: Same as Meal 1.

MEAL 6: 8 ounces grilled chicken breast, 1 cup brown rice, 1 cup steamed broccoli.

MEAL 7 [optional]: Same as Meal 1.

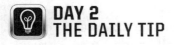 **DAY 2**
THE DAILY TIP

To get the best results from your diet, you have to watch everything you eat. Purchase a kitchen scale and a set of good measuring cups, and measure and weigh everything that goes into your mouth. You may be surprised at what amount actually constitutes a "serving."

DAY 3 WHEN YOU HIT ROCK BOTTOM

I had accomplished just about everything I set out to do in competitive bodybuilding. My titles include Mr. America (now known as the NPC Nationals), Mr. Universe, Professional Mr. World, 1st Arnold Schwarzenegger Classic Champion, and too many others to list here. Sure I had some professional disappointments. Three times I was runner up for the biggest and most coveted title in professional bodybuilding—Mr. Olympia. But if you come in second place to Lee Haney, a true freak of nature and a longtime friend and workout partner of mine, you still have a lot to be proud of if you know you did your best. And I knew I did.

It was 1993. Injuries had caught up with me and my professional career was clearly over. I had opened a gym that was bleeding money—and it wasn't like I had made a lot of money as a professional body builder in the first place. I hadn't really prepared myself for the transition from being a competitor to being a businessman. I hadn't dug very deep on how to set up a business plan. I didn't know the real costs of running a business. I think I assumed that my work ethic and optimistic spirit would be enough. The number at the bottom of my combined personal and business balance sheets was shrinking faster than I could think. I needed to get out from under owning the gym but couldn't find a buyer. Things quickly went from bad to worse. To my great embarrassment, I went bankrupt.

There I was—34-years-old and moving back home to live in my mom and dad's house—starting over. I felt sorry for myself—but not for long. That's not how I was raised. I got my game face on and began the slow and painful process of rebuilding. I worked as a trainer and sold supplements on the side. Because of my years as a bodybuilder and all I had learned first-hand and through my voracious study of nutrition, I started working with a supplier on developing my first custom supplements—I believed it was time to upgrade the industry. After seven or eight months I was definitely picking up some momentum in rebuilding my finances and my new business. I began to see a light at the end of the tunnel. It wasn't long before I expanded my operations from the basement and took over Mom's garage, too. It served as my warehouse. That may not sound like much to you—but I was darn proud of progress.

But then one day my mom's house caught on fire due to an electrical problem and burned completely to the ground. Thank God she had insurance to cover rebuilding the house and replacing her belongings. But I lost all my competition memorabilia and my entire supplement inventory—which was uninsured. Before you shake your head and roll your eyes, just remember I already told you I hadn't made the transition to businessman yet! I know better now. I look back and laugh at myself now—but it was no laughing matter at the time. I had gone from the frying pan to the fire!

I'm going to finish the story of how I built my business later—it's a good one—and tell you what I did to rebuild yet again. But here is what I want to plant in your mind right now. It's my definition of a winner. A winner in my book is someone who gets back up after he or she has been knocked down. Even if he has to live in his mom's basement and it only gets worse from there, if he gets back up, he's a winner. A loser stays down. A winner gets back up no matter how many times he or she is flat on the ground.

I am such a positive, energetic person that people are surprised to find out the number of setbacks I've had. When you are smiling on the cover of a magazine it doesn't tell the story of injuries and other hardships. I have a lot to be proud of, but if there's one thing I would brag about, it isn't the highest moments in my life, it is the fact that I got back up in the lowest moments.

Are things tough for you right now? Does it feel like you have hit rock bottom in life? Not sure you want to get back up? Do you feel defeated physically before you've even given this program a chance?

I don't want to make light of tough times for anybody but the old adage is true: When you hit the bottom there's no place else to go but up.

But there's another quote that is even more important: Victory is never final; defeat is never final.

You can still be a winner. All you have to do is get back up. It happens in that second. Even as you raise you win. That's what I did when I hit rock bottom and I know you can, too!

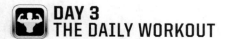

DAY 3
THE DAILY WORKOUT

THE MUSCLE BUILDER: LEGS
(Take 45 seconds - 1 minute rest between each set)
Lying leg curls – 5 sets of 10-12 reps
Stiff-legged deadlifts – 4 sets of 10-12 reps
Leg extensions – 5 sets of 10-12 reps (double drop set on last set)
45-degree Leg Press – 4 sets of 15 reps (double drop set on last set)
Hack Squat – 3 sets of 15 reps (triple drop set on last set)
Superset: Squats, walking lunges – 3 sets of 15-20 reps

CARDIO
20-30 minutes interval cardio on treadmill

HARDGAINER WORKOUT: REST

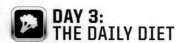

DAY 3:
THE DAILY DIET

MEAL 1: Myofusion Shake: 2 scoops Myofusion, 1/2 cup egg whites, 2/3 cup instant oatmeal, 1 tablespoon natural peanut butter or almond butter, 1/2 cup apple juice, 1/2 cup water and ice.
MEAL 2: Myofusion Protein Pancakes: 1 scoop Myofusion, 1 cup egg whites, 1 cup oatmeal, 1/4 cup chopped walnuts, 1 sliced banana. Mix all together and cook on low heat on a non-stick pan using cooking spray. Optional: add sugar-free syrup.
MEAL 3: Same as Meal 1.
MEAL 4: Egg omelet: 1 cup egg whites mixed with 1 cup chopped peppers, onions, and tomatoes. 1 slice watermelon on the side.
MEAL 5: 10 raw almonds.
MEAL 6: 8 ounces mahi mahi or other white fish, 1 small potato, 3 ounces steamed string beans, 4 ounces green salad with vinegar.
MEAL 7 *(optional)*: Same as Meal 1.

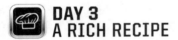

DAY 3
A RICH RECIPE

MYOFUSION MUFFINS

1 scoop MyoFusion Protein (any flavor)

1 whole egg OR egg white

Water

Mix egg and MyoFusion powder in a smallbowl, adding a little water at a time until it reaches the consistency of cake batter. Scoop batter into a small muffin-size cup and cook in the microwave for 30 seconds to one minute.

The muffin should rise like a cake would. If the muffin looks wet, keep adding 10 seconds until muffin is formed. This simple recipe will give you about 40 grams of protein and 8 carbs.

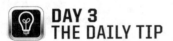

DAY 3
THE DAILY TIP

Keep your diet when you're on the road! It doesn't have to be as hard as people make it out to be. It begins with a decision to make good food choices. Grilled chicken with a baked potato and a green salad with just a drizzle of dressing can take the place of any suggestions you see throughout this book. I always order chicken, fish or lean steak and still stay on track with my intake.

DAY 4 THE RIGHT PEOPLE IN THE RIGHT PLACE

This may come as a surprise to you—and I don't recommend it for professional bodybuilders—but it was fine for me. I never had a coach.

Now that's not to say I accomplished everything on my own. My parents were great and I grew up in a home with a lot of love and support—even if my dad did think this bodybuilding thing I got into was crazy. I also had the wisdom I picked up from the bodybuilding greats that went before me. I soaked up everything my heroes like Joe Weider and others wrote. Heck, I even bought the Charles Atlas program from an ad in a comic book! I was the skinny kid that didn't want sand kicked in my face. If it had to do with building muscle, I read it.

But I was a bit of a loner. I didn't do team sports. My parents were immigrants to this great country. My dad didn't have the background or knowledge to take me out in the yard to toss a baseball or have me go out for passes while he winged a football at me. We didn't have a basketball net in the driveway. I wasn't tall enough for a basketball career anyway. But Dad gave me my work ethic and I think that was the greatest lesson any kid could have learned.

It was when I was twenty that I packed up my few belongings, loaded them into one of my dad's old beat up suitcases, and flew to Southern California, the mecca of bodybuilding. It was there I was offered a job by Ed Connors, the owner of Gold's Gym. He saw the potential in me and made me a manager of Gold's in Reseda, California.

Things started happening—which is usually the case when you work hard. Lee Haney saw my ferocious intensity from across the weight room and asked me to be a training partner. He is the one who taught me to work smarter. I was bench-pressing 525 pounds as part of a normal workout. He showed me how to stimulate muscles instead of destroying them by using less weight and better form.

My point is simple. Even for a guy like me who likes to do things on his own, we all need the right people around us. The best relationships are mutual, where both parties push, compliment, and help the other improve. I honestly believe I helped Lee as much as he helped me. I know he would agree with that statement.

This isn't just a lesson for bodybuilding. Nowhere is it more true than in business. One of my greatest sources of pride as the owner of Gaspari Nutritional Systems is being vendor of the year for both GNC (five times) and Vitamin King. I've done everything in Gaspari Nutrition from helping to develop and test new formulas to packing boxes to making sales calls and promotional appearances. I've mopped the floors a few times, too. But believe me, I know I couldn't have done any of this without hiring— and occasionally firing—the right people.

Who do you have on your team? Are they making you better? Are you making others better?

How many times have we seen a kid with all the potential in the world but they get caught up with the wrong friends, the wrong group, and his or her life goes the wrong direction?

If you train with people who practice bad form and give mediocre effort, you aren't nearly as likely to give your ultimate effort to achieve your ultimate body. If your best friends on the job do nothing but complain and have a terrible work ethic, you probably aren't doing your career any favors. Hang around people with lousy attitudes and don't be surprised to discover you have a lousy attitude too.

You've picked up this book and started this program for a reason. Not just to do a little better. But to do a lot better—to have your *ultimate* body. Surround yourself with the right people—people who help you and who you can help. Grow together. Encourage and push each other. Be each others' fans and hold each other accountable to better effort for better results. If you absolutely can't find the right workout partners, or the colleagues to help you grow in your chosen career, then at minimum make a commitment to stretch your mind and vision through select books and videos. Study what the greats do and follow their lead.

Count me as a member of your team. I believe you can accomplish more than you think. Believe in it yourself and surround yourself with people who will help you reach your goals and great things will happen.

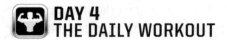

DAY 4
THE DAILY WORKOUT

THE MUSCLE BUILDER: SHOULDERS & ABS
(Take 45 seconds - 1 minute rest between each set)

Seated barbell front press – 4 sets of 8-12 reps
Giantset: Seated side laterals, Arnold Press, Standing dumbbell upright rows – 4 sets of 10-12 reps
Incline one arm side laterals – 3 sets of 12-15
Machine rear laterals – 4 sets of 12-15
Barbell shrugs from behind – 4 sets of 12-15
Twisting crunches – 4 sets of 30 reps
Leg raises – 4 sets of 25 reps

CARDIO
20-30 minutes interval cardio on treadmill

HARDGAINER WORKOUT: CHEST/BACK/BICEPS/TRICEPS/ABS
Modified Compound Superset #1
Flat Dumbbell Bench Press: 3 sets of 8, 6, 4 reps (90 second rest)
Close Grip Neutral Grip Pull-Ups: 3 sets of 8, 6, 4 reps (Strap weight on if you can – 2 minutes rest)

Note: If you cannot perform the Close Grip Pull-Up, either have someone spot you by using your legs off their hands for leverage or have them spot-push you up by the waist. There is also the chin assist machine if your gym has it.

Modified Compound Superset #2
Incline Barbell Bench Press: 3 sets of 8, 6, 4 reps (90 second rest)
Bent Over Underhand Barbell Row: 3 sets of 8, 6, 4 reps (2 min rest)
Giant Modified Compound Super Set #3 – *Take prescribed rest between exercise*
Chest Dips: 3 sets of 8, 6, 4 reps (60 second rest)
Preacher Curls: 3 sets of 8, 6, 4 reps (45 second rest)
Close Grip Bench Press: 3 sets of 8, 6, 4 reps (2 min rest)
Giant Modified Compound Super Set #4

E-Z Preacher Curls: 3 sets of 8, 6, 4 reps (60 second rest)
Lying Triceps Extensions: 3 sets of 8, 6, 4 reps (45 second rest)
Swiss Ball (aka "Inflated Fitness Ball") Crunches: 3 sets of 20, 15,
    10 reps (Hold a weight plate or dumbbell overhead if you can)
    (2 min rest)

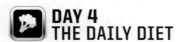 **DAY 4
THE DAILY DIET**

MEAL 1: Myofusion Shake: 2 scoops Myofusion, 1/2 cup egg whites,
    2/3 cup instant oatmeal, 1 tablespoon natural peanut butter or
    almond butter, 1/2 cup apple juice, 1/2 cup water and ice.
MEAL 2: Myofusion Protein Pancakes: 1 scoop Myofusion, 1 cup egg
    whites, 1 cup oatmeal, 1/4 cup chopped walnuts, 1 sliced
    banana. Mix all together and cook on low heat on a non-stick
    pan using cooking spray. Optional: add sugar-free syrup.
MEAL 3: 10 raw almonds.
MEAL 4: 8 ounces grilled chicken breast, 1 cup brown rice, 1 banana.
MEAL 5: Same as Meal 1.
MEAL 6: 8 ounces lean ground beef, 1 cup gluten-free pasta,
    4-6 ounces low sodium natural tomato sauce with 1
    tablespoon grated cheese [optional], 4 ounces green salad
    with vinegar.
MEAL 7[optional]**:** Same as Meal 1.

DAY 4 FOOD NOTE
On the road, if I don't have a blender, I do 2 scoops of Myofusion mixed with water and apple juice. I also have a handful of almonds and 3 or 4 rice cakes.

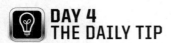 **DAY 4
THE DAILY TIP**

Shoulder injuries, in my opinion, are the most common among bodybuilders. I suggest warming up with laterals and rotations using light dumbbells to help prevent this.

DAY 5 *OH, THE PLACES YOU'LL GO!*

The first time I visited Russia on a business trip in the late 90s, I found out I was an "underground" star, with my popularity dating back to the era of the Soviet Union. I also learned that any obstacles I had to being a bodybuilder were nothing compared to the conditions in the Eastern Bloc. Why? Simple answer. Bodybuilding was against the law. You read that right. It was deemed by the Communist Party to be an individualistic sport that contributed nothing to society. I'll admit bodybuilding is an individual pursuit, but history has already judged Communism's view of collectivism. I also know that the growth of bodybuilding has been part of and contributed to the growth of an overall fitness emphasis in America. So I have no apologies and plenty of pride.

Powerlifting was a huge sport in the Soviet Union. Legends like Vasily Alekseyer—who set 80 world records and won Olympic gold in Munich and Montreal—were "rock stars" and party favorites. Any athlete who brought the USSR glory in the Olympics or other international events was revered. And while I admire athletes in this sport tremendously and recognize their almost superhuman strength, let's face it—the great power lifters didn't exactly have lean, ripped physiques. It wasn't uncommon for the best to have huge stomachs that looked bloated.

But with Perestroika and the breakup of the Communist Bloc, I became the first professional bodybuilder to appear on the cover of a Russian publication.

Legally that is.

Bodybuilding has grown exponentially in Russia over the past two decades and my business has had a strong footprint there since the late 90s. I travel to Moscow, St. Petersburg, and other cities to do promotional appearances and conduct business almost every year.

Why do I tell you all this? I am still amazed that a kid from Edison, New Jersey, the son of Italian immigrants, who barely left the state during his first twenty years, and got around mostly by bicycle or public transportation, has now travelled the globe many times.

I don't say this to brag, but I am humbled at how far I have come and where life has taken me as I have strived to reach my goals as a bodybuilder—overcoming both big and small setbacks along the way. Heck, I had "arrived" in the Soviet Union as an underground icon long before I actually got to the country in person. I feel a little bit like the character in Dr. Seuss' children's book, *Oh, the Places You'll Go!* And I know I'm not done travelling to new places.

I mean that both literally and metaphorically.

I want you to work this program and reach your goals in achieving your ultimate body. But I also want you to know that you will experience other successes in your life through this process of setting a goal and working your butt off to achieve it. You may never travel to Russia—and maybe you don't want to. But I bet you'll be amazed at the places this program will take you. Don't just take my word for it—read Dr. Seuss' classic if you need more convincing and encouragement.

Okay, enough daydreaming today. Push yourself hard. Do that and the success spillover will take care of itself. It may not come in the exact form you are expecting, but enjoy the surprise rewards that will be yours.

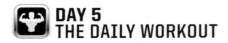

DAY 5
THE DAILY WORKOUT

THE MUSCLE BUILDER: BICEPS & TRICEPS
(Take 45 seconds - 1 minute rest between each set)

Superset: Incline dumbbell curls, Rope pushdowns—4 sets of 10 reps

Superset: Standing barbell curls, Seated 2-arm overhead tricep extension with dumbbell—4 sets of 10 reps

Superset: Seated preacher curls with EZ curl bar, Lying pullover press—4 sets of 10 reps

Superset: Dumbbell concentration curls, cable kickbacks— 4 sets of 10 reps

CARDIO
20-30 minutes interval cardio on treadmill

HARDGAINER WORKOUT: THIGHS/HAMSTRINGS/DELTS/CALVES
Modified Compound Superset #1

Medium Stance Squats: 3 sets of 12, 10, 8 reps (90 second rest)

Lying Leg Curls: 3 sets of 12, 10, 8 reps (90 second rest)

Note: If you suffer from lower back problems you may substitute the squat for the leg press. Since you are performing the leg press as your second exercise, then just use a close stance on this one and a medium stance on the second one.

Modified Compound Superset #2

Leg Press: 3 sets of 8, 6, 4 reps (90 second rest)

Barbell Romanian Dead-lifts: 3 sets of 15, 12, 10 reps (2 min rest)

Modified Compound Superset #3

Seated Barbell Front Shoulder: 3 sets of 10, 8, 6 reps (60 second rest)

Standing Calf Raise (Gastrocs): 3 sets of 10, 8, 6 reps (2 min rest)

Modified Compound Superset #4

Dumbbell Lateral Raises: 3 sets of 8, 6, 4 reps (60 second rest)

Lying Leg Raises with a pop at the top of each rep: 3 sets of 20, 15, 12 reps (60 second rest)

Descending Set #5—*Drop the weight as you move from set-to-set.*

Seated Calf Raises (Soleus)—3 Descending Sets: Decrease weight as you descend, if necessary:
- 1st set of 12-15 reps (15 sec rest)
- 2nd set of 12-15 reps (15 sec rest)
- 3rd set of 12-15 reps (1 min rest & repeat 2 more times)

DAY 5 WORKOUT NOTE
In leg training I feel more leg contraction when at the top of the movement. I fully flex my leg and squeeze!

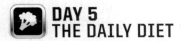

DAY 5
THE DAILY DIET

MEAL 1: Myofusion Shake: 2 scoops Myofusion, 1/2 cup egg whites, 2/3 cup instant oatmeal, 1 tablespoon natural peanut butter or almond butter, 1/2 cup apple juice, 1/2 cup water and ice.

MEAL 2: Myofusion Protein Pancakes: 1 scoop Myofusion, 1 cup egg whites, 1 cup oatmeal, 1/4 cup chopped walnuts, 1 sliced banana. Mix all together and cook on low heat on a non-stick pan using cooking spray. Optional: add sugar-free syrup.

MEAL 3: Same as Meal 1.

MEAL 4: 6 ounces lean buffalo patty *(or 93% lean ground beef)* with salsa or mustard, 1 cup brown rice, 6 ounces green salad with vinegar.

MEAL 5: 4 brown rice cakes.

MEAL 6: 8 ounces grilled chicken breast, 1 sweet potato, 1 cup asparagus.

MEAL 7 *(optional)*: Same as Meal 1.

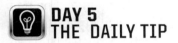

DAY 5
THE DAILY TIP

I do dumbbell curls on a bench differently than most people. First, I like to set the incline at about 30 degrees. Second, I don't twist the dumbbell on the way up. I keep it straight. I feel the most muscle contraction that way.

DAY 6 PUSH HARDER

I'm known in the world of bodybuilding and fitness as "The Dragon Slayer." I was one of the youngest men in the history of the sport to turn pro back in 1984 just after I won the IFBB World Amateur Championships at the age of 21. As a pro, I set a new standard in conditioning and became the first man to ever display striated glutes.

What you may not know is that I was never "supposed" to succeed as a bodybuilder. Even when I started competing, people tried to tell me I had no future in the sport. It's true that my genetics were less than perfect—though I'm going to clarify that later in the book. Believe me, I'm not apologizing for what I was born with. But in my sport I knew there would always be guys out there that were bigger, taller, and wider than me—with more naturally gifted structures. I couldn't do a thing about any of that. But I decided it didn't matter. What I did have was a will to be the best and the resolve to make it happen. I wanted it more than anybody else did, and I would do whatever it took to win. If I had to train harder than any other man on the planet, so be it. If I had to be more meticulous with my diet than all the other guys, fine. Nothing and no one was going to stop me. No one I saw was going to push harder than me. I know that for a fact. Because if I did see someone who was particularly intense, I used that as motivation to beat him in the gym.

During my pro career, I became famous for two things: my shredded condition, and my almost inhuman training intensity. I am proud to say that whenever there are discussions or debates about who the hardest-training bodybuilder of all time is, my name is always mentioned at the top of the list along with legends like Tom Platz and Dorian Yates. You see, I figured out very early on that one of the few things I could absolutely control was how hard I pushed in the gym. I wasn't afraid of hard work, and I definitely didn't shy away from pain or discomfort. Instead, I welcomed them and sought them out each and every time I walked onto the gym floor. When the sets got tough, I was just getting started. I would take my workouts into places almost no other bodybuilder dared to go, or had the guts to try for. In my mind, every workout was do or die. There were no "light days," and I never saw the gym as a social club to hang out and chit-chat. I was in there for one reason and one reason only, to test myself against that cold iron and give it everything I had.

You may dream about having a better physique. You may get discouraged at times because you don't know if you'll ever have a body you can be proud of. You stare at the pictures of the guys in the magazines and they look like they're aliens from another planet. What's it going to take for you to have a physique that's dense with thick muscle, one that looks chiseled out of granite? I'm talking about the type of muscles you don't want to hide—and you wouldn't be able to even if you tried. What if I told you that the absolute most important factor in turning that vision into flesh and blood is nothing more than your attitude? Once you decide that you are going to push harder every day, to put forth more effort than you thought possible or that anybody else thought you were capable of, nothing can stop you.

The guys and girls that sit around wishing they had exceptional bodies will never have them. The ones that aren't willing to do what it takes every day will always be average, nothing special at all. But the ones who push harder to reach their goals and refuse to listen to the voices inside and outside their heads telling them they can't do it—you'd better believe they will make it happen.

What is the gym to you? Is it just a building with a bunch of weights and machines? Or is it a foundry where you forge your physique in the fires of intensity? Most people just go to the gym to work out. They may want to look good, but they don't want to have to work too hard. A lot of their time is spent resting, talking to their buddies, and checking out the other members. They are more concerned with their hairstyle and outfit than actually training. Yeah, they go through the motions, but they stick to pretty easy stuff and don't often break a sweat. If you ask, they have a million excuses why they aren't as big or strong as they'd like to be.

Remember the old cliché, "No Pain, No Gain?" Learn to live by that mantra. Most people never build an extraordinary physique because they can't handle the pain, and they stop their sets before they've really stimulated any growth. Think about it for a minute. What's the most painful body part to train? That's easy—legs. There are few things you will ever do in life that are as excruciating as a 20-rep set of squats, drop sets of leg extensions, or super-setting hack squats and lunges. It literally feels like there is battery acid melting your muscles down to the bone. Squats are the worst. Your lungs feel like they are going to burst and your head may just explode from the pressure. Not many guys can take that kind of pain. Not many guys have great legs either. That's no coincidence.

If you want to look better than the average Joe in the gym, you have to push harder. There's no other way.

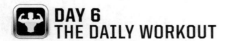 **DAY 6**
THE DAILY WORKOUT

THE MUSCLE BUILDER: REST

HARDGAINER WORKOUT: REST

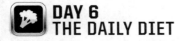 **DAY 6**
THE DAILY DIET

MEAL 1: Myofusion Shake: 2 scoops Myofusion, 1/2 cup egg whites, 2/3 cup instant oatmeal, 1 tablespoon natural peanut butter or almond butter, 1/2 cup apple juice, 1/2 cup water and ice.

MEAL 2: Myofusion Protein Pancakes: 1 scoop Myofusion, 1 cup egg whites, 1 cup oatmeal, 1/4 cup chopped walnuts, 1 sliced banana. Mix all together and cook on low heat on a non-stick pan using cooking spray. Optional: add sugar-free syrup.

MEAL 3: Same as Meal 1.

MEAL 4: 6 ounces grilled chicken breast, 1 cup brown rice, 1 apple.

MEAL 5: 10 raw almonds.

MEAL 6: 8 ounces baked salmon, 1 cup quinoa, 3 ounces steamed string beans, 4 ounces green salad with vinegar.

MEAL 7 *[optional]*: 2 scoops Myofusion, 1/2 cup apple juice, 1 tablespoon natural peanut butter or almond butter, 1/2 cup water and ice.

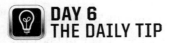 **DAY 6**
THE DAILY TIP

Being Italian, I love to have my Italian dinner at least once a week— usually on Sunday. You can have one meal of pure pleasure a week and still keep a great diet.

DAY 7 THE SECRET TO SUCCESS

Getting your ultimate body is hard work. You have to work on your diet. You have to take your intensity up to a level you haven't reached before and train like a wild beast. Going to the gym is serious business and I want you to be like me when you are there. I want you to leave nothing on the gym floor.

But I have a secret for you that is incredibly simple and a whole lot easier than monitoring your diet and working out like a warrior. Don't miss this. I know a lot of hard-core bodybuilders already know this—but forget or ignore it and it catches up with them when it's show time. I think you already know the secret too—but if you are like countless others I have trained and counseled you don't think it's a big enough deal to act on. It may be easy, but it's still overlooked at every level of bodybuilding and fitness training. Are you ready? Can you handle it? Can you take it on with the same sense of urgency and importance as you do your workout? *You have to rest.*

You have to make recovery a priority. It's not just a nice break from the action. It's not optional. It's an imperative. You have to take days off from the gym—and you have to get your sleep. In fact, I would argue that ignoring the need for sleep is having a devastating effect on our society at large. I have a friend in the medical profession who swears America is going to kill itself due to lack of sleep.

When I showed up in Venice Beach, California, let me

tell you, the opportunities to go out and have a good time were every-where. It wasn't always easy to go home and hit the sack when others were going out, but I knew I had to let my body heal. When it came time to compete, I destroyed guys who had a lot more natural size and ability than I had. Why? They worked hard in the gym, but then they went out and partied all night. I know a lot of young people feel it's their duty to hit the clubs a couple nights a week. There's an even bigger temptation to do that as you see your body start to change. You get leaner and more muscular and you want to get out in the scene and show your stuff.

Unlike what you see on TV, being like one of the guys on *Jersey Shore*—and growing up there I can tell you it's a real lifestyle—will not make you a champion. You won't reach your goals.

I'm not your dad and I can't tell you what to do. I don't want to. But I can tell you that your body is not made to be pushed to its limit and not be given a chance to rest. That's why I've scheduled two days off for those who are reading this book and working the program to really get big and ripped. For those looking to add impressive muscle but want an overall leaner appearance, I've given you a workout schedule that requires taking three days off. Lowering your intensity on workout days so you can add another workout isn't going to give you what you want. Get in the gym, go like an animal, then get out of there just like I've laid out for you.

When it comes to sleep—you have to get your eight hours. When I made the jump at age 22 to be a professional bodybuilder, I knew I needed my sleep. Lee Haney taught me how to get the most out of my workout without destroying my muscles. But no one had to tell me to get to bed at a reasonable hour and let my body recover. Everything I've learned in my career has simply been a confirmation of what I already intuitively knew. Sleep does two things for you. It lets your muscles heal from the beating you've given them in the gym, allowing them to get bigger, leaner, harder, and more defined. But it also lets you recharge your batteries so that you don't slouch into the gym for your next work-out. Instead, you can go in there with determination on your face, ready to make an assault on the weights.

I get a lot of credit from my peers for having the absolute best work ethic they've ever witnessed. I'm proud of that. But what a lot of people don't realize about my approach to bodybuilding is that I was just as serious about resting. Days off were days off. Nighttime was for sleep. I even took a solid nap of about an hour every afternoon to make positively sure my body was getting all the rest it needed. I can guarantee you that if I had run around all night like everyone else I would have accomplished next to nothing as a bodybuilder. And I doubt very much I would be the owner and CEO of a $100 million supplement company.

Let me add here that rest just isn't for bodybuilders and fitness fanatics. It is for business men and women; it is for stay-at-home moms; it is for students—and yes, I know how tempting it is to stay up studying late at night all week and then hit the clubs and parties all weekend. But no one is at their best without proper rest. It's simply not how we were created. There's a time to work, a time to play, and a time to rest.

Now I said this was a secret that is simple and easy. But bad habits get ingrained and changing them can be a challenge. Start where you are. Add a thirty minute catnap if that helps—and make getting more sleep at night a priority.

On your day of rest do something special with your loved ones—wife, children, significant other, friends. I recommend you get outside and play a game or take a hike. It keeps you well rounded—and you don't get tired of the gym. It also keeps those who are special to you satisfied.

Tonight, turn off the computer, the television, the stereo, and even the smartphone—and get under the covers and close your eyes. If there's stuff you didn't get done today, don't worry about it right now. Get your sleep and you'll get more done tomorrow—in life and in the gym.

Life is all about choices. You can choose to be like all the other young guys and run around until sunrise, or you can sleep and give your muscles adequate opportunity to repair the damage you've inflicted on them so you can keep growing bigger and better. Always remember that you stimulate growth in the gym, but you grow outside of it. Being diligent about getting the rest you need between workouts is the only way those intense training sessions will ever bear fruit in the form of massive biceps, triceps, pecs, lats, quads, hams, delts, and calves. You simply can't build your ultimate body without proper rest.

Now you know the secret. What are you going to do with it? Why not hit the sack early tonight and sleep on it.

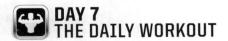

DAY 7
THE DAILY WORKOUT

THE MUSCLE BUILDER: REST

HARDGAINER WORKOUT: REST

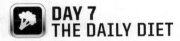

DAY 7
THE DAILY DIET

MEAL 1: Myofusion Shake: 2 scoops Myofusion, 1/2 cup egg whites, 2/3 cup instant oatmeal, 1 tablespoon natural peanut butter or almond butter, 1/2 cup apple juice, 1/2 cup water and ice.

MEAL 2: Myofusion Protein Pancakes: 1 scoop Myofusion, 1 cup egg whites, 1 cup oatmeal, 1/4 cup chopped walnuts, 1 sliced banana. Mix all together and cook on low heat on a non-stick pan using cooking spray. Optional: add sugar-free syrup.

MEAL 3: Same as Meal 1.

MEAL 4: 8 ounces grilled chicken breast, 1 cup brown rice, 1 cup steamed broccoli.

MEAL 5: 10 raw almonds.

MEAL 6: Egg omelet: 1 cup egg whites mixed with 1 cup chopped peppers, onions, and tomatoes. 1 slice watermelon on the side.

MEAL 7 [*optional*]**:** Same as Meal 1.

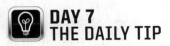

DAY 7
THE DAILY TIP

Sleep is the best weapon for building your ultimate body and ultimate health. Aminos are an important recovery tool, but nothing beats rest. Do whatever you have to and make room in your schedule for at least eight hours each day.

DAY 8 NO MORE EXCUSES

I know that I'm not a competitive bodybuilder anymore. But that doesn't mean I can't train like a competitor. If there's one thing I've learned, it's that I still can push myself to look like I am ready to get back on stage.

One of the greatest things about my 51-day journey to getting my ultimate body back was the reaction of others. Every day I brought a cooler to the office filled with the meals I had prepared ahead of time. I s cheduled my meetings around my workouts. I've always done some workout—but it had never been a big enough priority before to move business meetings around as needed. People couldn't help but notice how strict my routine had become.

Then there was the obvious physical transformation. My body started getting harder, my abs were getting more definition by the day, my arms and chest were gaining size, my veins were getting bigger. Nobody said anything, but I knew people were watching me closely.

Then, about a month into it, someone who works with me finally blurted out in a meeting, "Yeah, Rich is coming back. The Dragon Slayer is going to compete again!" I laughed and let everyone know that wasn't happening. But I was working so hard that some still were convinced I was on my way to the stage again. They weren't the only ones. The bodybuilding media was buzzing about a comeback. I'll say more about that later.

When I started posting my progress on Twitter and

Facebook to let my friends know what I was up to, that set off a whole new round of speculation.

"Admit it," a good friend said to me, "you are making a comeback to compete."

"You want the truth?" I asked him.

"I know the truth," he said. "You want to compete again."

"Well, you're probably right," I said. "I'd love to compete. But I'm 48—and I'm not going back on stage. That's not what this is about."

"Then what?" he asked. I finally had his attention.

"I got tired of making excuses for not having the body I wanted to have. It's always something: 'I'm too busy with the company. My kids are growing up so fast and my family needs me. I'm getting older.' All of those things may be true—and I'm going to take care of my business, my family, and be comfortable with myself at whatever age I am. But I wanted to say to myself and millions of others—there's no excuse for not getting into shape."

That didn't put rumors inside my company and within the body-building world to rest right away, but now, almost a year after starting this journey, I think people finally believe me—that I did this for myself. But most of all, I hope they hear my message that life is too short to make excuses.

Now that doesn't mean that you and I can control everything. Stuff happens. There can be injuries or illness. Work really can be demanding. Having a family takes energy and commitment too. Let's face it, we can tell our kids we love them all we want, but a kid spells love with four different letters: T-I-M-E.

So I recognize that life comes at us fast and furious. But I still won't back down on saying that there are no excuses for not getting into shape. You don't have to follow my ideal of the perfect body. I'm a get-ripped, get-big bodybuilder at heart. But you need to strive for your ideal of what you believe your ultimate body is. Why am I reminding you of that? I don't want you to use, "I can't look like Rich Gaspari," as an excuse. That's fine and good. I want you to look like *you* at your very best.

I've trained with enough people to know that we can hear something, but not necessarily internalize it. You may know in your head that even if circumstances aren't ideal, there are no more excuses for you to not get into shape. But it might not be deep down in your heart and soul yet. If that's the case, I want you to take a notecard or small sheet of paper and write down every excuse you can think of for why you can't achieve your ultimate body. Carry it with you to your next couple of workouts. Look at it. Read it over and over. And when you know for sure you aren't going to let any of those excuses get in the way at the gym; on your diet; of your rest—I want you to burn that piece of paper to symbolize your commitment to prevail no matter what.

Because you and I both know the truth. There are no more excuses for not getting in great shape.

DAY 8
THE DAILY WORKOUT

THE MUSCLE BUILDER: CHEST & ABS
(Take 45 seconds - 1 minute rest between each set)
Incline dumbbell press—4 sets of 8-10 reps
Incline dumbbell flies—4 sets of 8-10 reps
Decline cable flies—4 sets of 8-10 reps
Superset: Dumbbell flat bench, Pec Dec—4 sets of 8-10 reps
Crunches—4 sets of 25-30 reps
Leg raises—4 sets of 25-30 reps

CARDIO
20-30 minutes interval cardio on treadmill

HARDGAINER WORKOUT: CHEST/BACK/BICEPS/TRICEPS/CORE
Modified Compound Superset #1—*Take 45 seconds rest before moving on to the 2nd exercise*
Incline Dumbbell Press: 3 sets of 4-6 reps (45 Sec Rest)
Barbell Bent Over Row: 3 sets of 4-6 reps (1 min rest)
Modified Compound Superset #2 – *Take 45 seconds rest before moving on to the 2nd exercise*
Flat Dumbbell Bench Press: 3 sets of 6-8 reps (45 Sec Rest)
Chin-Ups: 3 sets of 6-8 reps (Strap on weight if you can)(1 min rest)
   Note: If you cannot perform the Chin-up, either have someone spot you by using your legs off their hands for leverage or have them spot-push you up by the waist.
Superset #3—*No rest between exercises*
Barbell Curls: 3 sets of 8-10 reps (No Rest)
Close Grip Dumbbell Bench Press (Triceps): 3 sets of 8-10 reps (1 min rest)
Superset #4—*No rest between exercises*
Dumbbell Hammer Curls: 3 sets of 10-12 reps (No Rest)
Triceps Pushdowns: 3 sets of 10-12 reps (1 min rest)
Superset #5—*No rest between exercises*
Plank: 2 sets of 1 Minute Static Contraction (No Rest)
Bicycle Maneuver: 2 sets of 30 reps (1 min rest)

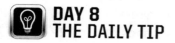

DAY 8
THE DAILY DIET

MEAL 1: Myofusion Shake: 2 scoops Myofusion, 1/2 cup egg whites, 2/3 cup instant oatmeal, 1 tablespoon natural peanut butter or almond butter, 1/2 cup apple juice, 1/2 cup water and ice

MEAL 2: Myofusion Protein Pancakes: 1 scoop Myofusion, 1 cup egg whites, 1 cup oatmeal, 1/4 cup chopped walnuts, 1 sliced banana. Mix all together and cook on low heat on a non-stick pan using cooking spray. Optional: add sugar-free syrup.

MEAL 3: Same as Meal 1.

MEAL 4: 8 ounces grilled chicken mixed with 1 cup brown rice, 1 tablespoon olive oil or salad dressing with 1 cup fresh veggies.

MEAL 5: Same as Meal 1.

MEAL 6: 8 ounces lean ground beef, 1 cup gluten-free pasta, 4-6 ounces low sodium natural tomato sauce with 1 tablespoon grated cheese *[optional]*.

MEAL 7 *[optional]*: Same as Meal 1.

DAY 8
THE DAILY TIP

If your ab muscles tend to hide—try doing an ab workout in every training session to complement whatever body areas you are hitting that day.

DAY 9 DO IT FOR YOU

The first cover I did for *Iron Man* magazine was in 1988—
as the hero, *Hercules Incarnate*. My last cover shoot was
the April 1992 edition—or so I thought. I never dreamed I
would be featured on a cover 20 years later. I think I felt
like a 20-year-old kid again when I got the October 2011
issue in the mail with me—now 48-years-old—on the
cover. And I looked pretty good, I have to admit. How in the
world did this come about?

I was inducted into the Muscle Beach Hall of Fame on
Memorial Day weekend, 2011. While I was there, I ran into
John Balik, the owner of *Iron Man*. We caught up a little
and then he asked me if I would ever consider appearing
on a cover again.

"I'd love to," I said quickly.

"Good," he said, "we have an opening and the photo
shoot is on July 15. Can you be ready?"

My mind started doing the math as quick as I could.
That would give me 52 days to prepare for a photo shoot.
Could I do it? At age 48?

"You bet I can," I answered. That's how I've always
been. Accept the challenge and figure out how to get it
done later.

I mentioned up front that I was still in good shape. You
have to be if you own a nutritional supplement company.
People would tell me I looked good. But a lot of people
would add, "Not like you used to look, but good."

So I knew I had serious work to do to be ready. I was

eating four meals a day—I had to ratchet that up to seven immediately. I was training four days a week—that increased to five. No way was I going to miss any training opportunity.

That's the mechanics of what I did. But what drove me? Was it to promote my company? Sure. But we were growing nicely already. Nothing as crazy as what I did was necessary!

Was it to avoid embarrassing myself on a magazine cover with nothing but posing shorts on? I don't think so. But who knows? Pride can be a great motivator.

I thought back to the last *Rocky* movie that came out in 2006, *Rocky Balboa*. There's a scene where Rocky is asked why he's making a comeback and he says, "I still have the fire in my belly. I'm doing it for me." I like that. And that is my real reason. I did this program for me.

There may be a lot of thoughts and motivations swirling around in your head. Maybe you are trying to get someone to notice you. Maybe you want to show your parents what you can accomplish. I've been there, too. But let me say to you right now: do it for you. For your own personal sense of accomplishment. I'm a people pleaser. You may be too. That's fine. Nothing wrong with it. But don't forget the one person you are with 24 hours a day, the one you see in the mirror each morning. And here's a little secret you probably already know: when you please yourself you are usually more pleasing to those around you. It's almost impossible to impress yourself and not impress others. If you want to take care of the important people in your life better, start by taking better care of yourself.

Recommit yourself to this program. Hit the gym with a passion today. Don't do it for Rich Gaspari. Do it for you . . . impress *yourself*!

DAY 9
THE DAILY WORKOUT

THE MUSCLE BUILDER: BACK & CALVES
(Take 45 seconds - 1 minute rest between each set)
Deadlifts—4 sets of 8-10 reps
Wide grip chins—4 sets of 8-10 reps
Superset: Close grip pulldowns, wide grip cable pullovers
    —4 sets of 8-10 reps
Superset: Cable low rows, T-bar rows—4 sets of 8-10 reps
Superset: Two arm dumbbell rows, machine rows—4 sets of 8-10 reps
Standing Calf raises—5 sets of 15 reps
Seated calf raises—5 sets of 15 reps

CARDIO
20-30 minutes interval cardio on treadmill

HARDGAINER WORKOUT: THIGHS/HAMSTRINGS/DELTS/CALVES/LOWER ABS
Superset #1 Wide Stance Squats: 3 sets of 4-6 reps (45 Seconds Rest)
Stiff Legged Barbell Deadlifts: 3 sets of 4-6 reps (1 min rest)
> Note: Utilize the "Full Body Tension Technique": This is when you
> stay in proper anatomical form and maintain that posture by
> keeping all of your major muscles contracted before & throughout
> the movements – This will keep you safe, while allowing you to use
> maximum intensity.

Giant Set #2—*3 exercises performed back-to-back without rest*
Leg Press: 3 sets of 6-8 reps (No Rest)
Leg Extensions: 3 sets of 10-12 reps (No Rest)
Lying Leg Curls: 3 sets of 10-12 reps (1 min rest)
Giant Set #3
Upright Barbell Row: 3 sets of 8-10 reps (No Rest)
Lateral Raises: 3 sets of 8-10 reps (No Rest)
Descending Set #4—*Drop the weight as you move from set-to-set*
Standing Calf Raises (Gastrocs) - 3 Descending Sets – Decrease weight
    as you descend, if necessary:
    • 1st set of 12-15 reps (15 sec rest)

- 2nd set of 12-15 reps (15 sec rest)
- 3rd set of 12-15 reps (1 min rest & repeat 2 more times)

Superset #5

Bent Over Lateral Dumbbell Raises: 3 sets of 10-12 reps (No Rest)
Seated Calf Raises (Soleus): 3 sets of 10-12 reps (1 min rest)
Hanging Leg Raises: 3 sets of 15-20 reps (1 min rest)

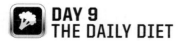 ## DAY 9
THE DAILY DIET

MEAL 1: Myofusion Shake: 2 scoops Myofusion, 1/2 cup egg whites, 2/3 cup instant oatmeal, 1 tablespoon natural peanut butter or almond butter, 1/2 cup apple juice, 1/2 cup water and ice.

MEAL 2: 1 cup steel cut oatmeal sprinkled with ground cinnamon and 1/2 cup fresh blueberries.

MEAL 3: Same as Meal 1.

MEAL 4: 8 ounces grilled chicken mixed with 1 cup brown rice, 1 tablespoon olive oil or salad dressing with 1 cup veggies.

MEAL 5: Myofusion Protein Pancakes: 1 scoop Myofusion, 1 cup egg whites, 1 cup oatmeal, 1/4 cup chopped walnuts, 1 sliced banana. Mix all together and cook on low heat on a non-stick pan using cooking spray. Optional: add sugar-free syrup.

MEAL 6: 8 ounces broiled mahi mahi or other white fish, 1 small potato, 3 ounces steamed string beans, 4 ounces green salad with vinegar.

MEAL 7(optional)**:** Same as Meal 1.

DAY 9 FOOD NOTE

Mix up your recipes. I like to swap bananas for blueberries or raspberries or both in the recipes I give you. I sometimes replace walnuts with natural peanut butter and mix it with chocolate Myofusion. (Yum!) I'll keep saying it: come up with your own recipes to build variety.

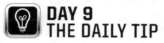 ## DAY 9
THE DAILY TIP

Form is very important on lateral raises. Raise the dumbbells out to the sides, making sure your elbows are higher than your forearms. As you raise the weights, turn your wrists toward the front and put all the tension on the side heads. Imagine that you're slowly pouring water out of two pitchers.

DAY 10 IRON SHARPENS IRON

At the age of 21, I was ready to take another step forward in my bodybuilding career. My plan was to drop a weight class and compete as a light heavyweight to make a run at the Nationals the following year. I had moved to California, the epicenter of bodybuilding, and taken fifth in my first national event.

As I mentioned earlier, I had caught the attention of Ed Connors who offered me a job managing a Gold's Gym. I was also working as a personal trainer on the side to make some extra cash. Even with two jobs, I wasn't making a lot of money, but I was young and single and didn't really need that much to get by. I was happy with where my life was and had no complaints. But then I lost my roommate and couldn't afford my apartment. I moved out in a hurry and there was about a week when I hadn't found a permanent spot to live. I slept in my car one night and crashed at different friends' places for a couple more nights while I was looking for something I could afford.

Just as all this was happening, Lee Haney asked me to become his regular training partner and help him get ready for Mr. Olympia. After we worked out one day, I told him what was going on. He did something incredible, one of the nicest things anyone has ever done for me. He offered me the spare bedroom at his house in Woodland Hills. I knew he was a great guy, but that's when I discovered this gentle giant from Atlanta, Georgia, was maybe the nicest guy in the world. Lee's wife, Shirley, was also amazing. It couldn't have been easy to have a loud kid from Jersey move into her home, but she was always gracious and kind. If she wanted to kill him for inviting me into their home, she never let me know it!

I still remember Lee's exact words: "You'll live in my home and we'll train."

Someone once read me a quote by King Solomon from the Bible that says, "As iron sharpens iron, so one person sharpens another," [Proverbs 27:17]. It may have been Lee. He's a very spiritual person. I'm no scholar, but I have to tell you, when I think back on this time in my life, I understand why Solomon was considered a wise man. Put two tough guys together and they both get tougher.

Lee was already a professional at the time. It was obvious he was going to be a major force in the world of bodybuilding. When I moved in, he was getting ready for the 1984 Mr. Olympia in New York City. It was his second try at the title. Did it work out great for us as training partners? You bet. Did we always get along? That's another story.

For example, I'm a morning person and Lee wasn't. That wouldn't have been a problem except for the fact that I love to sing in the shower. The truth is I'm not very good—but I do love to sing! Lee needed his rest. And the walls were thin. There were more than a few occasions when I know Lee wanted to kill me! That ended my singing career.

But his kindness, generosity, and tolerance were well rewarded when he won his first Mr. Olympia that year. He went on to win that competition an unprecedented streak of eight straight times, breaking Arnold Schwarzenegger's record of seven total wins. They say records are made to be broken, but I didn't think anyone would ever come close to what Lee had done. But then Ronnie Coleman came along and matched Lee's feat with eight straight wins of his own.

Would Lee have won in 1984 without me? There's a good chance he would have, but he'll be the first to tell you that my workout ferocity helped him reach new levels in his training. Frankly, he didn't have to work out as hard as me. But I think I pushed him to be his best.

Iron sharpens iron.

The same could be said for me. Would I have achieved what I did without Lee? Maybe. We'll never know. I can say that Lee taught me more about bodybuilding on a practical level than anyone else I know.

He was the first one to tell me I had to cut back on the amount of weight I was pushing—525 pounds on the bench press and close to 900 pounds in squats at the time.

"Stimulate your muscles, don't annihilate them," he always told me. He taught me to train like a bodybuilder instead of like a power-lifter. I learned to do full-range motions from Lee. I would watch the precision with which he would squeeze those muscles and stimulate them to growth. To be honest, I don't think I could have pulled off my 51-day transformation at age 48 if I hadn't learned that principle from Lee. I had plenty of injuries as it was, but my body could never have held up under the wear and tear of the way I used to train.

When I see Lee now, I still always say to him, "Thank you for all you taught me and did for me. Without that I could never have competed against you. It's because of you that I came as close as I did to beating you."

Iron sharpens iron.

You don't have to have a coach or a training partner like Lee Haney to reach your goals. But I would still encourage you to keep your eyes open for help from those around you. Who is going to push you when your motivation isn't at its peak? Who is going to hold you accountable to your goals and not let you make excuses? That's the kind of training partner you want to have in the gym. It's the kind of business colleague you want working at your side. It's the kind of friendship you want to build your social life around. Why?

Iron sharpens iron.

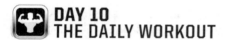
DAY 10
THE DAILY WORKOUT

THE MUSCLE BUILDER: LEGS
(Take 45 seconds - 1 minute rest between each set)
Lying leg curls—5 sets of 10-12 reps
Stiff-legged deadlifts—4 sets of 10-12 reps
Leg extensions—5 sets of 10-12 reps (double drop set on last set)
45-degree Leg Press—4 sets of 15 reps (double drop set on last set)
Hack Squat—3 sets of 15 reps (triple drop set on last set)
Superset: Squats, walking lunges—3 sets of 15-20 reps

CARDIO
20-30 minutes interval cardio on treadmill

HARDGAINER WORKOUT: REST

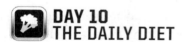
DAY 10
THE DAILY DIET

MEAL 1: Myofusion Shake: 2 scoops Myofusion, 1/2 cup egg whites, 2/3 cup instant oatmeal, 1 tablespoon natural peanut butter or almond butter, 1/2 cup apple juice, 1/2 cup water and ice.

MEAL 2: Myofusion Protein Pancakes: 1 scoop Myofusion, 1 cup egg whites, 1 cup oatmeal, 1/4 cup chopped walnuts, 1 sliced banana. Mix all together and cook on low heat on a non-stick pan using cooking spray. Optional: add sugar-free syrup.

MEAL 3: Same as Meal 1.

MEAL 4: 8 ounces grilled chicken breast, 1 cup quinoa, 1 cup steamed broccoli.

MEAL 5: 10 raw almonds.

MEAL 6: 8 ounces of lean steak, 1 sweet potato, 1 cup raw kale salad with 1 teaspoon olive oil and lemon juice.

MEAL 7 *(optional)*: Same as Meal 1.

DAY 10 FOOD NOTE

If you're tired of me mentioning shakes, consider that my shortcut to success on my diet. You have to eat but honestly, I don't have a big appetite. Shakes are easy for me to get the protein and other nutrients I need. If you're tired of them, substitute in an egg white omelet and add veggies and Ezekiel bread for carbs.

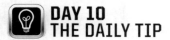

DAY 10
THE DAILY TIP

Excuse: I don't see any results. **Answer:** *Intensity and patience. Rome wasn't built in a day, so you shouldn't expect your body to transform in a week. If your training regiment is spot-on and you aren't cutting corners, try covering up for a bit and assess your progress every two weeks or so. When you look in the mirror, you'll be pretty blown away by what you see!*

DAY 11 COMPETITION IS A GOOD THING

I don't know what age kids should be when we start keeping score in youth soccer or baseball or football or whatever. I don't believe seven-year-olds need a Vince Lombardi-style coach. The idea is that kids need to be encouraged to participate in sports and healthy activities and have fun while they are doing it. I agree.

But there does come a point in time when we need to keep score and not just give everyone a trophy for simply showing up. Bullying, taunting, and demeaning trash-talk are not appropriate at any age and shouldn't be tolerated. But by the time we hit the preteen and teen years, we need to know when we've succeeded and when we've come up short. We need to start learning the lessons of competition. Kids are smart. They don't want something shiny that says they did something great when they know they didn't do very well. Competition is how we find out how we're doing. It's a good thing. Even when we are disappointed. We live, we get over it, we get better.

My first time on stage was in 1979. It was just a local bodybuilding meet and most of the guys who competed in it were from the same gym. I had started lifting like crazy by the time I was fourteen but I didn't feel like I was ready. I entered on a dare. You see there was a guy one year older than me who had been in some competitions and brought home some medals. Other kids took him seriously. He was admired. Me? I was just a gym rat.

I thought to myself, *I can beat this guy.* I knew I was a

lot stronger—I hadn't arrived yet, but I was well on my way to benching 400 pounds and squatting 600 pounds as part of my workouts in high school! But it wasn't the lack of respect from my peers that got me to take that dare to compete for the first time—it was Paul himself.

In the gym one day, Paul let me know I was nothing compared to him. After all, he had "competed." That was a mistake on his part. He woke the sleeping dragon inside of me. I no longer just thought I could beat him—I was determined to beat him. I registered for Physique '79.

I came in 6th place. Not a very auspicious start. It would take me three more years to not only win the youth section of the event—but the overall as well. But here's the good news: I beat Paul. Hey, you can laugh—because I sure did—but that competition showed me I still had a long way to go to become a champion. At the same time, beating Paul gave me the confidence to believe I could achieve what I set out to do.

Competition is good. It pushes us to do better than what we think we are capable of. It lets us know where we fall short. I won plenty of hardware in my career. But I never captured the greatest prize in bodybuilding—Mr. Olympia. I always had a mountain named Lee Haney blocking my path. I didn't have the genes to produce the freakish width of his clavicles or his naturally narrow waist. I knew there was only one way in the world I was going to beat him. I was going to have to outwork him.

Even I cringe when I think of some of my workouts back then—I basically doubled what everyone else was doing and did two sessions a day. Why? I wanted to beat Lee. I never got him in Mr. Olympia, but competing against him pushed me to achieve levels of greatness I would never have approached otherwise. I've told Lee that I thought that there was at least one year and maybe two that I thought I really did have him beat. He laughs and tells me I might be right—but the trophy is staying at his house. To become a champion, you have to beat the champion—and in a judged competition, it can't be just by the narrowest of margins. You have to be the clear winner. I couldn't do that, but I still reached new heights by trying with everything I had in me.

The lesson I learned is that the greatest competition you can face is when you go up against yourself. When Usain Bolt runs the 100 m or 200 m and sets a new world record, is he competing against the field or himself? Since no one is within three strides of him, the only way he can get better is to compete against himself. Did the late Steve Jobs, the legendary CEO of Apple, sit in his office all day worrying about how he could beat Bill Gates? I'm sure the two men felt some personal competition. But if Steve had spent all his time thinking about Bill, he wouldn't have had so many breakthroughs where he bested what he had done before. He competed with himself.

Let me dare you. It's time for you to get up on that stage—in whatever venue of your life that you need a challenge. It's time for you to show how far you've come. Here's who you have to beat—*you!* You have to beat who you were when you were in the very best shape of your life. You have to beat you from a week ago and a month ago. And to get the trophy, you can't win by just a little. You have to show up and score a knockout victory. Are you up for the challenge? I know someone who says you can't do it. That person says you are nothing. They are planning to whoop you.

What are you going to do about it? Do you take the dare?

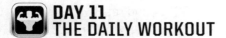

DAY 11
THE DAILY WORKOUT

THE MUSCLE BUILDER: SHOULDERS & ABS
(Take 45 seconds - 1 minute rest between each set)
Seated barbell front press—4 sets of 8-12 reps
Giantset: Seated side laterals, Arnold Press, Standing dumbbell
   upright rows—4 sets of 10-12 reps
Incline one arm side laterals—3 sets of 12-15
Machine rear laterals—4 sets of 12-15
Barbell shrugs from behind—4 sets of 12-15
Twisting crunches—4 sets of 30 reps
Leg raises—4 sets of 25 reps

CARDIO
20-30 minutes interval cardio on treadmill

HARDGAINER WORKOUT: CHEST/BACK/BICEPS/TRICEPS/ABS
Modified Compound Superset #1
Flat Dumbbell Bench Press: 3 sets of 8, 6, 4 reps (90 second rest)
Close Grip Neutral Grip Pull-Ups: 3 sets of 8, 6, 4 reps (Strap weight
   on if you can – 2 mins rest)
   *Note: If you cannot perform the Close Grip Pull-Up, either have
   someone spot you by using your legs off their hands for leverage
   or have them spot-push you up by the waist – and don't forget the
   chin assist machine.*

Modified Compound Superset #2
Incline Barbell Bench Press: 3 sets of 8, 6, 4 reps (90 second rest)
Bent Over Underhand Barbell Row: 3 sets of 8, 6, 4 reps (2 min rest)
Giant Modified Compound Super Set #3 – *Take prescribed rest
   between exercise*
Chest Dips: 3 sets of 8, 6, 4 reps (60 second rest)
Preacher Curls: 3 sets of 8, 6, 4 reps (45 second rest)
Close Grip Bench Press: 3 sets of 8, 6, 4 reps (2 min rest)
Giant Modified Compound Super Set #4

E-Z Preacher Curls: 3 sets of 8, 6, 4 reps (60 second rest)
Lying Triceps Extensions: 3 sets of 8, 6, 4 reps (45 second rest)
Swiss Ball (aka "Inflated Fitness Ball") Crunches: 3 sets of 20, 15,
    10 reps (Hold a weight plate or dumbbell overhead if you can)
    (2 min rest)

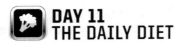 ## DAY 11
THE DAILY DIET

MEAL 1: Myofusion Shake: 2 scoops Myofusion, 1/2 cup egg whites,
    2/3 cup instant oatmeal, 1 tablespoon natural peanut butter
    or almond butter, 1/2 cup apple juice, 1/2 cup water and ice.
MEAL 2: Myofusion Protein Pancakes: 1 scoop Myofusion, 1 cup egg
    whites, 1 cup oatmeal, 1/4 cup chopped walnuts, 1 sliced
    banana. Mix all together and cook on low heat on a non-stick
    pan using cooking spray. Optional: add sugar-free syrup.
MEAL 3: Same as Meal 1.
MEAL 4: 8 ounces grilled chicken breast, 1 sweet potato, 1 cup
    steamed broccoli.
MEAL 5: Same as meal 1.
MEAL 6: 8 ounces baked salmon, 1 cup brown rice, 1 cup asparagus.
MEAL 7 *(optional)*: Same as Meal 1.

DAY 11 FOOD NOTE
I can eat the same thing every day. I know you don't want to hear that.
You may need more variety. There's a lot of mixing and matching you can
do to add variety. Rotate chicken, fish, turkey, and lean beef. Switch up
your carbs between mixed vegetables, Ezekiel bread, brown rice, yams,
potatoes, lentils, and a host of other great foods.

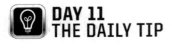 ## DAY 11
THE DAILY TIP

*Don't lace your fingers behind your neck when doing crunches. It puts
stress on your neck vertebrae.*

DAY 12 WRITE IT DOWN

The mind has been known to play tricks on each of us, particularly when it comes to memory. I had a fun "discussion" with a friend the other night about one of our early business meetings. I was positive we met at one restaurant and he was equally positive it was a different place. It was no big deal, but it illustrates how our memories get distorted over time—even the ones where we are absolutely certain we have right.

The best way to preserve your experiences accurately is a journal. Go into any Barnes and Noble, gift shop, or big box store, and you will find a nice array of journals. There are theme journals for moms, teens, wine lovers, book readers, travelers, leaders, teachers, and yes, for those who want to track their workouts. There are also online journaling programs and smartphone apps.

What do I use right now? I'm a self-directed, straight-forward kind of guy. I like a simple ruled journal. I don't want prompts on what to write. My journals for the past 30 years have been very task oriented.

What do I write? Simple.

- date
- meals
- supplements
- workout
- sleep
- results

The only guesswork in my journal is what shows up in the results section. Now if you are a pro bodybuilder, you do take measurements from time to time. You know what you can see in the mirror, but you need objective numbers, too. There was no guesswork for me on those days. I still remember the first time I measured 21-inch arms. I wrote it down. I knew precisely what areas were responding correctly to my regime and where I needed to put in some extra work. But I had been around the sport long enough that I could track my performance by what I saw in the mirror and how I felt.

You may be thinking, *Rich, I'm not sure I am that hardcore. That sounds like too much trouble.* No problem. I said from the very start that this program is about you—your dreams, goals, and needs. But I'll still encourage you to at least test journaling for a week. After seven days, read back over what you wrote. I know that's not long enough to gain deep insights on what works and what doesn't work long term. But you still might discover something there—and you might also find that you like keeping a record of your efforts and progress as much as I do.

At the very least, journaling offers a symbolic exercise that what you do each day is important. It all matters. It is worthy of being committed to paper. So write yourself a note that you can look back on in the future to see just how far you came once you set your mind to building your ultimate body!

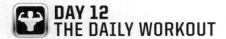

DAY 12
THE DAILY WORKOUT

THE MUSCLE BUILDER: BICEPS & TRICEPS
[Take 45 seconds - 1 minute rest between each set]
Superset: Incline dumbbell curls, Rope pushdowns – 4 sets of 10 reps
Superset: Standing barbell curls, Seated 2-arm overhead tricep extension with Dumbbell – 4 sets of 10 reps
Superset: Seated preacher curls with EZ curl bar, Lying pullover press – 4 sets of 10 reps
Superset: Dumbbell concentration curls, bench dips – 4 sets of 10 reps

CARDIO
20-30 minutes interval cardio on treadmill

HARDGAINER WORKOUT: THIGHS/HAMSTRINGS/DELTS/CALVES
Modified Compound Superset #1
Medium Stance Squats: 3 sets of 10, 8, 6 reps [90 second rest]
Lying Leg Curls: 3 sets of 10, 8, 6 reps [90 second rest]

Note: If you suffer from lower back problems you may substitute the squat for the leg press. Since you are performing the leg press as your second exercise, then just use a close stance on this one and a medium stance on the second one.

Modified Compound Superset #2
Leg Press: 3 sets of 12, 10, 8 reps [90 second rest]
Barbell Romanian Dead-lifts: 3 sets of 10, 8, 6 reps [2 min rest]
Modified Compound Superset #3
Seated Barbell Front Shoulder: 3 sets of 8, 6, 4 reps [60 second rest]
Standing Calf Raise (Gastrocs): 3 sets of 10, 8, 6 reps [2 min rest]
Modified Compound Superset #4
Dumbbell Lateral Raises: 3 sets of 10, 8, 6 reps [60 second rest]
Lying Leg Raises with a pop at the top of each rep: 3 sets of 10, 8, 6 reps [60 second rest]
Descending Set #5 – *Drop the weight as you move from set-to-set*
Seated Calf Raises (Soleus) - 3 Descending Sets – Decrease weight as

you descend, if necessary:
- 1st set of 12-15 reps [15 sec rest]
- 2nd set of 12-15 reps [15 sec rest]
- 3rd set of 12-15 reps [1 min rest & repeat 2 more times]

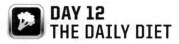

DAY 12
THE DAILY DIET

MEAL 1: Myofusion Shake: 2 scoops Myofusion, 1/2 cup egg whites, 2/3 cup instant oatmeal, 1 tablespoon natural peanut butter or almond butter, 1/2 cup apple juice, 1/2 cup water and ice.

MEAL 2: 8 ounces lean buffalo patty *[or 93% lean ground beef]* with salsa or mustard, 1 small potato, 6 ounces green salad with vinegar.

MEAL 3: Same as Meal 1.

MEAL 4: 8 ounces grilled chicken mixed with 1 cup brown rice, 1 tablespoon olive oil or salad dressing with 1 cup veggies.

MEAL 5: Same as Meal 1.

MEAL 6: Myofusion Protein Pancakes: 1 scoop Myofusion, 1 cup egg whites, 1 cup oatmeal, 1/4 cup chopped walnuts, 1 sliced banana. Mix all together and cook on low heat on a non-stick pan using cooking spray. Optional: add sugar-free syrup.

MEAL 7 *[optional]*: Same as Meal 1.

DAY 12 FOOD NOTE
For more flavor I use spray butter so food doesn't taste so bland.

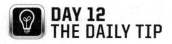

DAY 12
THE DAILY TIP

No doubt about it, big biceps are impressive. Start with standing barbell curl and watch your form. No swinging the back to help get the bar up. Then lower the bar slowly to maximize the rep.

DAY 13 YOU WILL NOT FAIL

I have already told you that after my bodybuilding career ended, I lost everything. The gym I owned. My entire savings. After the fire at my mom's house, my memorabilia, my inventory, and even the roof over my head was gone. I also told you that a winner is the man or woman who gets knocked down and gets back up.

For me, getting back up meant starting in yet another basement. Somehow that seemed fitting. My first workout room as a skinny 14-year-old kid who wanted to be like Arnold, was my parents' basement. As a 35-year-old who had lost everything, it was my mom's basement. After the fire, I moved into my brother's basement. It wasn't as nice as Mom's, but it was all I needed.

Did I have self-doubts? Sure. I had gone from a career that plastered me on TV screens and magazine covers with hundreds of thousands of fans to living off the generosity of family members. Was it time to get a "real" job and give up on this passion I still had for bodybuilding?

I actually hired on with an insurance company, went through their training program, and closed a sale on my first solo sales call. There's nothing wrong with being an insurance agent. But I knew it wasn't right for me. I wasn't done with bodybuilding. So I took the signed contract in to my boss, who was happy with me getting a sale, and I resigned. He wasn't as happy with that, but we had become friends and he understood I still had a passion for the world of bodybuilding. That doesn't mean that he and my family members didn't think I was a little crazy.

Maybe I was. After all, I still owed my supplement supplier $70,000. It felt like a fortune. But here's what I told myself: You will not fail.

It's hard to get new inventory when you haven't paid for the stuff that was destroyed in a fire. I made a promise to my supplier. I said, "I will pay you something every single week. Even if it's not much, I will pay you every cent." And I did. Why? Because I believed myself when I said, "You will not fail."

It doesn't matter if you don't have the job, the relationships, the body you want right now. Even if you've failed before, even if you are flat on your back right now—ultimately, you won't fail.

Get back up. Get in the gym. Move into your brother's basement if you have to. But most importantly, look yourself in the mirror and tell yourself, "You will not fail."

Words are powerful. Make sure your words are planting seeds of success and greatness in your life.

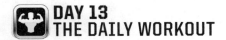
DAY 13
THE DAILY WORKOUT

THE MUSCLE BUILDER: REST

HARDGAINER WORKOUT: REST

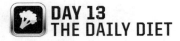
DAY 13
THE DAILY DIET

MEAL 1: Myofusion Shake: 2 scoops Myofusion, 1/2 cup egg whites, 2/3 cup instant oatmeal, 1 tablespoon natural peanut butter or almond butter, 1/2 cup apple juice, 1/2 cup water and ice.

MEAL 2: Myofusion Protein Pancakes: 1 scoop Myofusion, 1 cup egg whites, 1 cup oatmeal, 1/4 cup chopped walnuts, 1 sliced banana. Mix all together and cook on low heat on a non-stick pan using cooking spray. Optional: add sugar-free syrup.

MEAL 3: 10 raw almonds.

MEAL 4: 8 ounces grilled chicken, 1 cup quinoa, 1 cup grilled squash and zucchini drizzled with balsamic vinegar and 1 tablespoon olive oil.

MEAL 5: Same as Meal 1.

MEAL 6: Egg omelet: 1 cup egg whites mixed with 1 cup chopped peppers, onions, and tomatoes. 1 slice watermelon on the side.

MEAL 7 [optional]**:** Same as Meal 1.

DAY 13 FOOD NOTE
Everyone gets nervous when they hear the word "fats." But remember, essential fats are very important to keep the body healthy and actually speed up your metabolism.

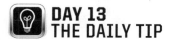

DAY 13
THE DAILY TIP

Your body has to have fat to burn fat. But make sure you are getting the right kinds of fat. With meat, I stick to grilled chicken, lean steaks, and fish. I get my essential fats from adding four grams of fish oil and eating my natural peanut butter and almonds.

DAY 14 A VOTE OF CONFIDENCE

Good things happened quickly for me once I went pro as a bodybuilder. *Wow, this is easy!* I thought as I started piling up the wins early and often. In my first Mr. Olympia contest, I took third place. I was only 22-years-old. That was unheard of. The only other man I know who did that well in his first Mr. Olympia was—you've probably already guessed it—Lee Haney.

A lot of people assume that my early success is what gave me so much confidence. With all honesty, I believe it was the opposite. I believe I had so much early success because I was so confident. Some of my friends and competitors back then described me as a brash, cocky Italian "kid" from Jersey. Some meant it as a compliment and others meant it to put me in my place.

But I think it went a lot deeper than just my smile and upbeat persona. I really did look at life positively. I was enthusiastic. It wasn't because everything had gone great for me and my family. When I was a young child, one of my older brothers died. I remember the house was filled with tears and mourning. We weren't poor, at least never in my eyes, but we were on that lower edge of the working middle class. So we didn't have the extras that so many people take for granted now.

So when I say that confidence brings success as much as success brings confidence, I say that with a realistic view of life. I know that life is a roller coaster and that there are ups and downs. But I've always believed—always known—that no matter what happens I am going to get back up, so the down times of life never defeated my buoyant optimistic spirit.

When you exude confidence, you tell the world you are a winner. When I was competing, I would go up on stage already believing I had won. It showed. I beat guys that were probably more naturally gifted than me physically. But I like to think I was more gifted than some of them in mental toughness and basic attitude. I was never into playing games to try to psyche somebody else out—but you know, I think my confidence did just that on more than a few occasions. I think my optimistic spirit allowed me to get absolutely every last scintilla of size and definition out of my body when I competed. I definitely ranked high in the intangibles of smile and personality.

How are you looking at life right now? Is the glass half-full or half-empty? Where are you on the roller coaster of life? In the deepest dip or at the top of the highest peak? It doesn't matter. What matters is your attitude. I believe the quality of life is determined more by our attitudes than our circumstances. We've all seen the guy who has absolutely everything going for him but still complains constantly. We've all seen the individual going through a tough time who still believes life is great. You might think I'm crazy, but I had just as much confidence when I lost everything I owned as I do now, when my company is soaring, and family are healthy and strong, and I'm in the best shape of my life.

If you feel like you are loser, you've already lost. If you feel like a winner, you've already won. Your outlook will impact everything from your workout in the gym, to your job, your relationships, and every other aspect of your life.

Rich, I don't feel like a winner right now.

I believe we all have choices and you can choose to have confidence. But it's not always easy and it comes more naturally for some than others. My advice right now is to fake it until you get it. I'm not suggesting you be loud and boastful. Some of the toughest people I've met as a bodybuilder and businessman have been quiet and humble. But when you feel like a winner, you can't hide it. Choose it, believe it, remind yourself of it, practice it, and it will come.

This 51 days to your ultimate body isn't just about your body, is it? You're going to acheive your ultimate *you!*

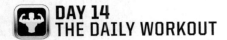

DAY 14
THE DAILY WORKOUT

THE MUSCLE BUILDER: REST

HARDGAINER WORKOUT: REST

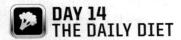

DAY 14
THE DAILY DIET

MEAL 1: Myofusion Shake: 2 scoops Myofusion, 1/2 cup egg whites, 2/3 cup instant oatmeal, 1 tablespoon natural peanut butter or almond butter, 1/2 cup apple juice, 1/2 cup water and ice.

MEAL 2: 1 cup steel cut oatmeal sprinkled with ground cinnamon and 1/2 cup fresh blueberries.

MEAL 3: Same as Meal 1.

MEAL 4: 8 ounces grilled chicken breast, 1 cup brown rice, 1 cup steamed broccoli.

MEAL 5: Same as Meal 1.

MEAL 6: 8 ounces of lean steak, 1 sweet potato, 1/2 cup mushrooms, 6 ounces green salad with vinegar.

MEAL 7 [*optional*]**:** Same as Meal 1.

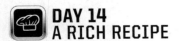

DAY 14
A RICH RECIPE

STEAK WITH MUSHROOMS

1/2 cup balsamic vinegar

1/2 cup red wine

2 cloves garlic, minced

1/4 cup low-sodium soy sauce

1 1/3 pounds lean flank steak

1 pound large shiitake mushrooms, stems removed

Freshly ground black pepper
1 tablespoon olive oil
Salt to taste

Combine first four ingredients to make the marinade. Brush half of the marinade on the flank steak, cover, and refrigerate for at least 30 minutes or overnight. In a separate bowl, toss the remaining marinade with the mushrooms, cover and refrigerate for 30 minutes or up to 2 hours.

Preheat grill to medium high. Remove the steak and mushrooms from the marinade and discard the marinade. Season the steak with salt and pepper. Brush the mushrooms with olive oil and season them with salt and pepper.

Grill the flank steak for 4 to 8 minutes on each side, depending on desired doneness. Grill the mushrooms for 3 minutes on each side. Let the steak rest for 1-2 minutes before slicing. Slice the steak and mushrooms on the bias. Arrange steak on a serving platter with the mushrooms on top. Serve warm.

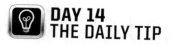

DAY 14
THE DAILY TIP

For variety I go for sashimi, brown rice and a green salad at my favorite Japanese restaurant. Like I always say, you can eat out when you make proper food choices.

DAY 15 TRY SOMETHING NEW

Follow the plan in this book as closely as you can and you will get a better body than you ever thought possible. As high as your expectations are—I think reality will beat them. But don't be afraid to try new things as well. Ideas come from all directions. There are so many incredible athletes today. Pay attention when they speak about their training. Watch closely when they show what they are doing on a video. Be ready to learn from everybody.

I devoured everything I could get my hands on when I started down the road as a bodybuilder. Joe Weider—the patron saint of bodybuilders. Charles Atlas—the guy who could turn anything from a chair to the floor into a sophisticated piece of exercise equipment—and who made sure the bully didn't kick sand in your face.

When the *Pumping Iron* documentary came out, I thought I was in heaven. This was before the days of home video rentals so I had to study the book. The only problem was when it first came out I didn't have enough money saved to buy a copy. When Arnold came to the mall nearby to sign copies, I rode my bike over and asked him to sign a sheet of paper I brought with me. I think I had actually read the entire book standing in the aisle of a bookstore before I was able to purchase it.

One of the things I was known for as a competitor was my striated glutes. That doesn't seem like a big deal now—all the top bodybuilders have striated glutes. But go back and look at champion bodybuilders through the years. Prior to my ascent in the mid 80s, no one else had this. There's a simple reason. I was one of the first guys to put lunges into my routine.

Now, at the time, lunges were considered a "girl exercise." If "girl exercise" was meant to be a slam, then the person saying it hasn't really done a true lunge. They also better not say that in front the top female athletes that are part of Team Gaspari. They might get their butt kicked. But one of the reasons I got those glutes was because I did walking lunges with really heavy weights—I might be holding 240 pounds in dumbbells—and then did the same with reverse lunges. I didn't really invent anything but I still came up with something brand new for male bodybuilders by keeping my eyes open to what was going on around me.

Another inspiration that I believe I brought not just to the bodybuilding community but all different forms of physical fitness was the superset. That's where you do a parallel workout on two body areas. You might do a set on the bench to work your chest and then rush over to the leg-lift machine and work your quads. You then rush back over to the bench and do your next set of presses. You basically work two body areas in the same amount of time as it takes to recover between sets doing just one area. You add intensity and get some cardio throughout your entire workout. I brought that approach from New Jersey to California with me. I was in one of the great gyms of the world with a who's who list of bodybuilders, and it didn't take long for others to adopt the practice.

The superset is pretty standard practice today and may not seem like a big deal now, but again, read through the old manuals and you won't find anything like it. Was it a brilliant idea on my part? Well, I think it was a pretty darn good idea, but my point is, I paid attention to what was being done and kept my mind and eyes open for better ways to do it.

These are two examples of my approach to bodybuilding. In my striving to be the best, I respected everything I could learn from others, but I knew myself so well, I was never afraid to try a new way of doing things to gain an edge.

I grew up in Edison, New Jersey, and our city was named after one of the great inventors of all time—Thomas Edison. He was the master of trial and error—and of taking technology that already existed and adapting it and synthesizing it with other technologies to come up with something entirely new and groundbreaking.

The lesson? Mix things up. Beg, steal, and borrow great ideas for improving your workout. But don't forget one very important source of new ideas and inspiration. You.

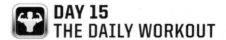

DAY 15
THE DAILY WORKOUT

THE MUSCLE BUILDER: CHEST & ABS
(Take 45 seconds - 1 minute rest between each set)
Incline dumbbell press – 4 sets of 8-10 reps
Incline dumbbell flies – 4 sets of 8-10 reps
Decline cable flies – 4 sets of 8-10 reps
Superset: Dumbbell flat bench, Pec Dec – 4 sets of 8-10 reps
Crunches – 4 sets of 25-30 reps
Leg raises – 4 sets of 25-30 reps

CARDIO
20-30 minutes interval cardio on treadmill

HARDGAINER WORKOUT: CHEST/BACK/BICEPS/TRICEPS/CORE
Modified Compound Superset #1 – *Take 45 seconds rest before moving on to the 2nd exercise*
Incline Dumbbell Press: 3 sets of 6-8 reps (45 Sec Rest)
Barbell Bent Over Row: 3 sets of 6-8 reps (1 min rest)
Modified Compound Superset #2 – *Take 45 seconds rest before moving on to the 2nd exercise*
Flat Dumbbell Bench Press: 3 sets of 6-8 reps (45 Sec Rest)
Chin-Ups: 3 sets of 6-8 reps (Strap on weight if you can)(1 min rest)

> *Note: If you cannot perform the Chin-up, either have someone spot you by using your legs off their hands for leverage or have them spot-push you up by the waist. (If you haven't figured it out by now, I love chin assist machines.)*

Superset #3 – *No rest between exercises*
Barbell Curls: 3 sets of 8-10 reps (No Rest)
Close Grip Dumbbell Bench Press (Triceps): 3 sets of 8-10 reps (1 min rest)
Superset #4 – *No rest between exercises*
Dumbbell Hammer Curls: 3 sets of 10-12 reps (No Rest)
Triceps Pushdowns: 3 sets of 10-12 reps (1 min rest)

Superset #5 – *No rest between exercises*
Plank: 2 sets of 1 Minute Static Contraction (No Rest)
Bicycle Maneuver: 2 sets of 30 reps (1 min rest)

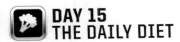 ## DAY 15
THE DAILY DIET

MEAL 1: Myofusion Shake: 2 scoops Myofusion, 1/2 cup egg whites, 2/3 cup instant oatmeal, 1 tablespoon natural peanut butter or almond butter, 1/2 cup apple juice, 1/2 cup water and ice.

MEAL 2: Myofusion Protein Pancakes: 1 scoop Myofusion, 1 cup egg whites, 1 cup oatmeal, 1/4 cup chopped walnuts, 1 sliced banana. Mix all together and cook on low heat on a non-stick pan using cooking spray. Optional: add sugar-free syrup.

MEAL 3: Same as Meal 1.

MEAL 4: Egg omelet: 1 cup egg whites mixed with 1 cup chopped peppers, onions, and tomatoes. 1 slice watermelon on the side.

MEAL 5: 10 raw almonds.

MEAL 6: 8 ounces mahi mahi or other white fish, 1 small potato, 3 ounces steamed string beans, 4 ounces green salad with vinegar.

MEAL 7 [*optional*]: Same as Meal 1.

DAY 15 FOOD NOTE
If you are craving variety and you haven't tried the Myofusion pancake recipe yet, now is the time!

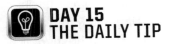 ## DAY 15
THE DAILY TIP

If you are adding mass for a competition you still need to be able to see your ab muscles. If you can't see them you are putting on too much fat.

DAY 16 JUST GO FOR IT

I'm still amazed that one of the biggest things that holds people back from getting into the gym, from seeking a promotion at work, from starting a business, from asking someone out, or from trying something new and challenging is the fear of failure, the fear of looking bad in the eyes of others. Maybe being born into a family with a father who knew he wanted something better and packed up his wife and firstborn to make the journey to America—with a detour through Canada on the way—instilled in me that you don't worry about what others think. You don't sweat it when there are obstacles and setbacks.

One of the most significant competitions in my life was the NPC Nationals in 1983 in San Jose, California. I was 208 pounds and I was competing in the heavyweight division. The lineup of bodybuilding greats I was competing against was incredible. These were my heroes. I had studied their pictures and read their training tips for years with the dream of someday being like them.

Rory Leidelmeyer came to Santa Monica as the clear favorite, but the winner ended up being Bob Paris, who is still a popular motivational speaker. Mike Christian, the legendary "Iron Warrior" took third place. Another great bodybuilder, Matt Mendenhall, took fourth place. In fifth place was a young kid out of New Jersey that no one had ever heard of before. His name was Rich Gaspari. My first competition as a teen I took sixth place, so believe me, on that stage, with those greats, I wasn't disappointed in taking fifth place. But I wasn't satisfied either. It only made me hungry for more. I can't tell you how excited I was to hear the key players in the bodybuilding industry talking about me as the guy to watch—and watch out for.

After the show, Ed Connors, the owner of Gold's Gym and my boss, came up to me and told me that if I would drop a weight class I could come back and win the NPC Nationals as a light heavyweight the next year. He was right. I dropped about 20 pounds and won my first national championship in 1984. What if I hadn't competed because I was too young and wasn't ready? What if I had been afraid of what others might think of me? Or if I had been too scared and intimidated to walk on stage to compete against some of my heroes? I certainly wouldn't have been in the position to win a championship the following year.

I'm not going to be a kinder and gentler trainer for you at this point. I don't care how awkward you feel about whatever it is you need to take on in life right now. What are you afraid of? Who cares what others think? You have a keg instead of six-pack around your middle and you don't want to look bad? So what. Of course you're not ready. But go for it anyway.

Ask her out. Tell your boss you want to be considered for a promotion. Sign up for a local competition. Get your butt kicked, learn, and win it next year!

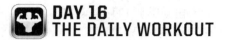 **DAY 16**
THE DAILY WORKOUT

THE MUSCLE BUILDER: BACK & CALVES
[Take 45 seconds - 1 minute rest between each set]
Deadlifts – 4 sets of 8-10 reps
Wide grip chins – 4 sets of 8-10 reps
Superset: Close grip pulldowns, Wide grip cable pullovers – 4 sets of
  8-10 reps
Superset: Cable low rows, T-bar rows – 4 sets of 8-10 reps
Superset: Two arm dumbbell rows, machine rows – 4 sets of 8-10 reps
Standing Calf raises – 5 sets of 15 reps
Seated calf raises – 5 sets of 15 reps

CARDIO
20-30 minutes interval cardio on treadmill

HARDGAINER WORKOUT:
THIGHS/HAMSTRINGS/DELTS/CALVES/LOWER ABS
Superset #1
Wide Stance Squats: 3 sets of 8-10 reps [45 Seconds Rest]
Stiff Legged Barbell Deadlifts: 3 sets of 8-10 reps [1 min rest]

> *Note: Utilize the "Full Body Tension Technique": This is when you
> stay in proper anatomical form and maintain that posture by
> keeping all of your major muscles contracted before & throughout
> the movements – This will keep you safe, while allowing you to use
> maximum intensity.*

Giant Set #2 – *3 exercises performed back-to-back without rest*
Leg Press: 3 sets of 6-8 reps [No Rest]
Leg Extensions: 3 sets of 10-12 reps [No Rest]
Lying Leg Curls: 3 sets of 10-12 reps [1 min rest]
Giant Set #3
Upright Barbell Row: 3 sets of 8-10 reps [No Rest]
Lateral Raises: 3 sets of 8-10 reps [No Rest]
Descending Set #4 – *Drop the weight as you move from set–to–set*

Standing Calf Raises (Gastrocs) - 3 Descending Sets – Decrease
weight as you descend, if necessary
  • 1st set of 12-15 reps (15 sec rest)
  • 2nd set of 12-15 reps (15 sec rest)
  • 3rd set of 12-15 reps (1 min rest & repeat 2 more times)
Superset #5
Bent Over Lateral Dumbbell Raises: 3 sets of 10-12 reps (No Rest)
Seated Calf Raises (Soleus): 3 sets of 10-12 reps (1 min rest)
Hanging Leg Raises: 3 sets of 15-20 reps (1 min rest)

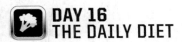 ## DAY 16
THE DAILY DIET

MEAL 1: Myofusion Shake: 2 scoops Myofusion, 1/2 cup egg whites, 2/3
cup instant oatmeal, 1 tablespoon natural peanut butter or
almond butter, 1/2 cup apple juice, 1/2 cup water and ice.
MEAL 2: Myofusion Protein Pancakes: 1 scoop Myofusion, 1 cup egg
whites, 1 cup oatmeal, 1/4 cup chopped walnuts, 1 sliced
banana. Mix all together and cook on low heat on a non-stick
pan using cooking spray. Optional: add sugar-free syrup.
MEAL 3: Same as Meal 1.
MEAL 4: 8 ounces grilled chicken, 1 cup brown rice, 1 apple.
MEAL 5: Same as Meal 1.
MEAL 6: 8 ounces lean ground beef, 1 cup gluten-free pasta,
4-6 ounces low sodium natural tomato sauce with
1 tablespoon grated cheese (optional).
MEAL 7 (optional): Same as Meal 1.

DAY 16 FOOD NOTE
I usually have apple juice, but as a change I mix orange juice with vanilla
Myofusion to create a creamy orangesicle flavor.

DAY 16
THE DAILY TIP

The one exercise I do just about every workout to work my calf muscles is the seated calf raise. It's about the only exercise designed to exclusively hit the soleus muscle.

DAY 17 YOU ARE WHAT YOU EAT

I've been asked a lot lately about how I got so ripped after all of these years of not competing. But the other big
question I get all the time is, how do I build solid, quality muscle? Without a base of good muscle, you're really
wasting your time dieting to get ripped up. You'll have abs,
but will you really look like you want to without the solid
quality muscle that goes with a ripped body? Probably
not.

A lean physique that has next to zero muscle mass is
hardly impressive. Before you get ripped, you need some
mass to show once the fat comes off. One phrase related to this I used to hear back in the day was "you can't
carve a twig!" So it's important to have enough muscle
that when you diet down you show good size in your chest,
back, shoulders, legs, and arms.

It takes several different tasks done simultaneously
to make it possible to build quality muscle. Possibly the
most overlooked component is nutrition. You want to
make sure you are gaining quality muscle and not just
getting fat and "bulking up." I have always said that if your
waist gets too thick and you lose sight of your abs, you're
way too fat. Of course, you can't stay totally ripped in the
process of gaining lean quality muscle either, so it's a fine
line you need to walk. I learned in my early years that bulking up too much caused me to have to diet too hard, to the
point where I ended up losing muscle. The best approach
is gaining a little at a time, so you are always able to see

your abs and some degree of detail in your body. Forget about trying to gain 30-40 pounds in a couple months. I guarantee most of it will be fat!

I have always felt the most important piece of the puzzle was eating. Following the right diet really matters. A lot of people say they eat great, but when I get down to seeing the details of their diet; they really don't. They are not eating the right percentages of their macronutrients, or eating frequently enough to keep the body in an anabolic state. I see many people saying they're eating right and taking in plenty of protein, but when it gets down to it they're eating four times a day at best. That's at least one meal shy of where they should be, and six or seven meals a day would be even better.

First, I recommend logging everything you are eating every day. Eat a diet that consists of 40% protein, 45% Carbohydrates and 15% fat, and split your daily food totals into at least six meals a day. This will seem impossible at first for most people. It takes planning! It's been said many times that if you fail to plan, you plan to fail. This definitely pertains to proper eating to gain lean muscle mass. The first thing to do is keep a diet log of everything you eat so you can see exactly whether or not you are following the right diet.

Before you do anything else, I recommend you write down everything you eat for the next three days to figure out how many calories you are taking in per day. When you figure this out, you can then take that caloric intake and follow more closely a 40%-45%-15% ratio diet by using a good book that states what the macronutrients of the foods are.

Make sure the foods you eat are high quality protein from chicken, lean beef, fish, egg whites, and some whole eggs plus protein powders like Myofusion. Carbohydrates will come from unrefined complex sources like rice, sweet potatoes, potatoes, oatmeal, gluten-free pasta, and gluten-free breads. I like to stay gluten-free lately since I feel I don't get as bloated or have as much water retention now that I have taken gluten out of my diet. I also eat fruits like bananas, apples, pears, strawberries, and blueberries. I eat fibrous carbs from vegetables like broccoli, string beans, spinach and other greens.

As you can see, I believe in a wide variety of food sources, but I like to stay away from the white sugars and white flour products. This way I gain quality weight in the form of muscle and not fat. My fats come from walnuts, almonds, whole eggs, fish oil, and olive oil. I stay away from fried foods as well, since these are empty calories that will not help in gaining muscle but will cause you to gain fat. This is the typical diet I follow to gain lean muscle mass, but you can change the diet to more or less of the proteins, carbs, and fats.

Gaining quality muscle is critical if you are going to achieve your ulimate body. Remember—you are what you eat. So make sure you give your body the right fuel that will build healthy muscle mass, not bulky fat.

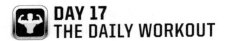

DAY 17
THE DAILY WORKOUT

THE MUSCLE BUILDER: LEGS
(Take 45 seconds - 1 minute rest between each set)

Lying leg curls – 5 sets of 10-12 reps
Stiff-legged deadlifts – 4 sets of 10-12 reps
Leg extensions – 5 sets of 10-12 reps (double drop set on last set)
45-degree Leg Press – 4 sets of 15 reps (double drop set on last set)
Hack Squat – 3 sets of 15 reps (triple drop set on last set)
Superset: Squats, walking lunges – 3 sets of 15-20 reps

CARDIO
20-30 minutes interval cardio on treadmill

HARDGAINER WORKOUT: REST

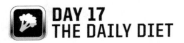

DAY 17
THE DAILY DIET

MEAL 1: Myofusion Shake: 2 scoops Myofusion, 1/2 cup egg whites, 2/3 cup instant oatmeal, 1 tablespoon natural peanut butter or almond butter, 1/2 cup apple juice, 1/2 cup water and ice.

MEAL 2: Myofusion Protein Pancakes: 1 scoop Myofusion, 1 cup egg whites, 1 cup oatmeal, 1/4 cup chopped walnuts, 1 sliced banana. Mix all together and cook on low heat on a non-stick pan using cooking spray. Optional: add sugar-free syrup.

MEAL 3: 10 raw almonds.

MEAL 4: 8 ounces grilled chicken, 1 cup quinoa, 6 ounces green salad with vinegar.

MEAL 5: Same as Meal 1.

MEAL 6: 8 ounces grilled tuna, 1 cup brown rice, 1 teaspoon of olive oil, 1 cup asparagus.

MEAL 7 *(optional)*: Same as Meal 1.

DAY 17 FOOD NOTE
Steamed chicken is delicious and has no extra cooking calories. Fat free spray dressings taste great and make it easier not to use too much on salads or meats.

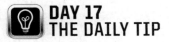 **DAY 17
THE DAILY TIP**

What quality foods should you be eating to get leaner and build muscle? Stock your pantry with the following "secret weapons" to help you increase your metabolism, burn fat, and improve the nutritional content of your diet:

- Kale
- Oats
- Vinegar
- Apples
- Avocado
- Lentils
- Blueberries

- Cinnamon
- Quinoa
- Salmon
- Almonds
- Green Tea
- Cayenne Pepper

DAY 18 A LITTLE RESPECT

I was afraid someone would pinch me and I would wake up. Sitting down across from Joe Weider and interviewing him for a Gaspari Nutrition video made me feel like a kid again. I knew I was in the presence of greatness. Here was a guy who built more than a personal media and nutritional and supplement empire. He created a whole industry.

Without Joe Weider, bodybuilding as we know it would not exist. He did tremendous things for my sport and for fitness at large. Now in his 90s, his voice wasn't as strong and clear as it had once been. But as always his words were powerful. Toward the end of our talk he said something that brought tears to my eyes. He said, "Rich, I'm proud of you and all you have accomplished, and I know this is just the beginning of all you are going to do."

This didn't happen when I was getting ready to go pro or at the height of my career. He said this after I had retired, hit rock bottom, and had finally gotten my lean and mean company up and running. He knew all the good things that I had pulled off, but he also knew the struggles I had, from injuries to going bankrupt. He was a friend to me the whole time. Some people who had accomplished a whole lot less than Joe wouldn't take my calls when I was down. He would. He was that kind of man. He cared about people. He built people up. And when he told me how proud he was of me, it felt like a confirmation that any hardships I had to overcome were worth it. He recognized that I was the same person in good times and bad—and

I was a fighter. Next to my dad, I can't think of anyone whose words of respect and blessing meant more to me.

So who exactly is Joe Weider? Joe is the man most responsible for the bodybuilding industry. He was big and strong but wasn't a body-builder himself. But he thought physical strength was important for a man's self respect. Back in the 40s and 50s, he was so far ahead of his time in understanding how supplements could maximize workout efforts. You'd better believe I was drinking his muscle milk as a teen-ager. He and his wife Betty—a pinup model and a pioneer for women's fitness—founded the International Federation of BodyBuilders (IFBB). With his brother Ben, he created Mr. Olympia and Ms. Olympia and other contests. He founded *Muscle & Fitness*, *Flex*, *Men's Fitness*, *Shape*, and other important magazines. When Arnold Schwarzenegger, then the governor of California, awarded Joe with the Venice Muscle Beach Life-time Achievement Award, he pointed out that it was Joe who inspired him to be a bodybuilder and immigrate to the United States.

There are literally millions who would say about the same thing, in-cluding a kid from Edison, New Jersey. I not only admired his accom-plishments, but I also admired that he did this starting at the bottom. He had $7 in his pocket when he launched his first company.

Respect is such an important theme to me. Self-respect. Respect from others. Respect for others. I am a firm believer that all of us have been created with infinite worth. But respect is something different from self-worth. It isn't something we are born with. It is both learned and earned.

I hope I have even a little of what Joe has—a genuine concern for people and a desire to see them reach for their dreams. This book is about a whole lot more than your ultimate body. It is about building the ultimate you. It is about learning to respect yourself and others respect-ing what you are accomplishing. The place to start is by showing more respect yourself. Our culture can be pretty cynical and negative. Get rid of that negativity. It won't take you anywhere.

But respect is one of those investments in life, where you end up receiving more than you give. Show it. Receive it. Live with it.

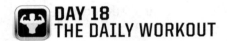

DAY 18
THE DAILY WORKOUT

THE MUSCLE BUILDER: SHOULDERS & ABS
[Take 45 seconds - 1 minute rest between each set]

Seated barbell front press – 4 sets of 8-12 reps

Giantset: Seated side laterals, Arnold Press, Standing dumbbell upright rows – 4 sets of 10-12 reps

Incline one arm side laterals – 3 sets of 12-15

Machine rear laterals – 4 sets of 12-15

Barbell shrugs from behind – 4 sets of 12-15

Twisting crunches – 4 sets of 30 reps

Leg raises – 4 sets of 25 reps

CARDIO
20-30 minutes interval cardio on treadmill

HARDGAINER WORKOUT: CHEST/BACK/BICEPS/TRICEPS/ABS

Modified Compound Superset #1

Flat Dumbbell Bench Press: 3 sets of 8, 6, 4 reps [90 second rest]

Close Grip Neutral Grip Pull-Ups: 3 sets of 8, 6, 4 reps [Strap weight on if you can – 2 mins rest]

> Note: If you cannot perform the Close Grip Pull-Up, either have someone spot you by using your legs off their hands for leverage or have them spot-push you up by the waist.

Modified Compound Superset #2

Incline Barbell Bench Press: 3 sets of 8, 6, 4 reps [90 second rest]

Bent Over Underhand Barbell Row: 3 sets of 8, 6, 4 reps [2 min rest]

Giant Modified Compound Super Set #3 – *Take prescribed rest between exercise*

Chest Dips: 3 sets of 8, 6, 4 reps [60 second rest]

Preacher Curls: 3 sets of 8, 6, 4 reps [45 second rest]

Close Grip Bench Press: 3 sets of 8, 6, 4 reps [2 min rest]

Giant Modified Compound Super Set #4

E-Z Preacher Curls: 3 sets of 8, 6, 4 reps [60 second rest]

Lying Triceps Extensions: 3 sets of 8, 6, 4 reps (45 second rest)
Swiss Ball (aka "Inflated Fitness Ball") Crunches: 3 sets of 20, 15, 10
   reps (Hold a weight plate or dumbbell overhead if you can)
   (2 min rest)

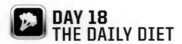 **DAY 18**
THE DAILY DIET

MEAL 1: Myofusion Shake: 2 scoops Myofusion, 1/2 cup egg whites, 2/3
     cup instant oatmeal, 1 tablespoon natural peanut butter or
     almond butter, 1/2 cup apple juice, 1/2 cup water and ice.
MEAL 2: 1 cup steel cut oatmeal sprinkled with ground cinnamon and
     1/2 cup fresh blueberries.
MEAL 3: Same as Meal 1.
MEAL 4: 8 ounces grilled chicken breast, 1 sweet potato, 1 cup grilled
     squash and zucchini drizzled with balsamic vinegar and
     1 tablsespoon olive oil.
MEAL 5: Same as Meal 1.
MEAL 6: 8 ounces of lean steak, 1 cup quinoa, 1 cup raw kale salad
     with 1 teaspoon olive oil and lemon juice.
MEAL 7 *(optional)*: Same as Meal 1.

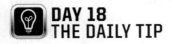 **DAY 18**
THE DAILY TIP

*Stretching between sets is great for ab workouts. Lay flat on your back
and stretch your arms as if you were reaching for something behind
you. Hold for 20 seconds.*

DAY 19 DO WHAT YOU LOVE

You can only become truly accomplished at what you love. So do what you love.

Why did I become a successful bodybuilder in the first place? After all, bodybuilding was a tiny little sport with very little exposure. How in the world did I build one of the finest nutritional supplement companies in the world—with little business background? Why did I throw myself back into a competition level training regime at age 48—and succeed?

Because I love it.

I've prospered more from the world of bodybuilding than I ever dreamed possible. But I didn't get into bodybuilding for the money. When I left Rutgers University after three years to see if I could go to the next level and be a pro, that wasn't a money grab. It was following my passion.

Do what you love. I think there are two great life lessons to take from that thought. The first might surprise you. But I believe we can actually fall in love with doing the right things. For example, almost everyone complains about eating right and following a disciplined diet. As I write this, I'm coming out of the holiday season, that time of year when there's tons of good food and friends—and lots of tempting desserts—all around us. But I stayed on my high protein, complex carbohydrates, gluten free, low sugar, healthy fat diet. Did I do this because of a promise I made to myself or because I had to? Nope. I stayed on my ultimate body diet because I've learned to love it.

If doing this program feels like a grind that doesn't have you excited, then it's time you clear your mind of negative thought patterns—yes, complaining and whining is often more a matter of habit than circumstances—and fall in love with the process of building your best body ever. Keep that internal transformation going outside the gym. If you are married, fall in love with your spouse all over again. If you are fortunate enough to have a job, be thankful and don't grouse about it when unemployment in the country is so high.

Now there is a second lesson to be learned from the statement *do what you love*. If you aren't growing and succeeding in life, you might be doing the wrong things. Hit your workout hard today. But also do some honest self-reflection. Have you truly pursued your passions in life? It's not about getting the most money or going with the crowd. It's about being true to yourself.

Don't consider this career counseling, consider it life counseling. Why settle for going through the motions? Life is a gift. An opporunity to be siezed and savored. It's time for you to stop settling.

Do what you love. That might mean you need to learn to love what is already right in front of you. If there's no way that's going to work, open your eyes, start paying more attention, do some digging, and go find what you were made to do.

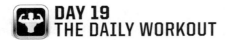

DAY 19
THE DAILY WORKOUT

THE MUSCLE BUILDER: BICEPS & TRICEPS
(Take 45 seconds - 1 minute rest between each set)

Superset: Incline dumbbell curls, Rope pushdowns – 4 sets of 10 reps

Superset: Standing barbell curls, Seated 2-arm overhead tricep extension with Dumbbell – 4 sets of 10 reps

Superset: Seated preacher curls with EZ curl bar, Lying pullover press – 4 sets of 10 reps

Superset: Dumbbell concentration curls, cable kickbacks – 4 sets of 10 reps

CARDIO
20-30 minutes interval cardio on treadmill

HARDGAINER WORKOUT: THIGHS/HAMSTRINGS/DELTS/CALVES

Modified Compound Superset #1

Medium Stance Squats: 3 sets of 8, 6, 4 reps (90 second rest)

Lying Leg Curls: 3 sets of 12,10, 8 reps (90 second rest)

Note: If you suffer from lower back problems you may substitute the squat for the leg press. Since you are performing the leg press as your second exercise, then just use a close stance on this one and a medium stance on the second one.

Modified Compound Superset #2

Leg Press: 3 sets of 10, 8, 6 reps (90 second rest)

Barbell Romanian Dead-lifts: 3 sets of 10, 8, 6 reps (2 min rest)

Modified Compound Superset #3

Seated Barbell Front Shoulder: 3 sets of 8, 6, 4 reps (60 second rest)

Standing Calf Raise (Gastrocs): 3 sets of 10, 8, 6 reps (2 min rest)

Modified Compound Superset #4

Dumbbell Lateral Raises: 3 sets of 10, 8, 6 reps (60 second rest)

Lying Leg Raises with a pop at the top of each rep: 3 sets of 10, 8, 6 reps (60 second rest)

Descending Set #5 – *Drop the weight as you move from set-to-set*

Seated Calf Raises (Soleus) - 3 Descending Sets – Decrease weight as you descend, if necessary:
  - 1st set of 12-15 reps (15 sec rest)
  - 2nd set of 12-15 reps (15 sec rest)
  - 3rd set of 12-15 reps (1 min rest & repeat 2 more times)

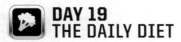

DAY 19
THE DAILY DIET

MEAL 1: Myofusion Shake: 2 scoops Myofusion, 1/2 cup egg whites, 2/3 cup instant oatmeal, 1 tablespoon natural peanut butter or almond butter, 1/2 cup apple juice, 1/2 cup water and ice.

MEAL 2: Myofusion Protein Pancakes: 1 scoop Myofusion, 1 cup egg whites, 1 cup oatmeal, 1/4 cup chopped walnuts, 1 sliced banana. Mix all together and cook on low heat on a non-stick pan using cooking spray. Optional: add sugar-free syrup.

MEAL 3: Same as Meal 1.

MEAL 4: 6 ounces canned tuna in spring water, 1 cup brown rice, 1 tablespoon olive oil or salad dressing with 1 cup veggies.

MEAL 5: Same as Meal 1.

MEAL 6: 8 ounces lean ground beef, 1 cup gluten-free pasta, 4-6 ounces low sodium natural tomato sauce with 1 tablespoon grated cheese *(optional)*.

MEAL 7 *(optional)*: Same as Meal 1.

DAY 19 FOOD NOTE
It's harder to find and more expensive, but consider adding buffalo to your diet. It is higher in protein and leaner than beef.

DAY 19
THE DAILY TIP

If you have to, carry a food chest or cooler to the office. People may think you're fanatical about your diet—but that's okay. The only way a busy person can eat seven meals each day is through careful planning and advance preparation.

DAY 20 DO YOUR HOMEWORK

Without a doubt, a large portion of my success as a professional bodybuilder was due to my use of supplements. To build the kind of muscularity necessary to compete in the sport of bodybuilding you have to give your body the right fuel. I'm not talking about steroids or other dangerous products—and believe me, I've been asked a thousand times during my career and even this transformation if I took any illegal stuff and the answer is always no. The supplements I am talking about are the right kind of proteins and probiotics to support massive growth.

When I first started bodybuilding as a young teen, the grocery store thought my mom was a professional baker. Why? I would go through a dozen eggs and at least a gallon of milk every day. I probably took for granted the cost of feeding me during those years and I'm sure there were more than a few times my dad wanted to put an end to my passion for bodybuilding just so he could afford to buy groceries. But then I almost pushed my mom over the edge when I saved up my money to buy Joe Wieder's Muscle Builder. She took me—and the powder I had bought—straight to the doctor to find out if this stuff was safe.

It was. Even back then I didn't do anything by guesswork. The supplement industry has come a long way since the dynamic days of Muscle Builder, but throughout my career I have stayed on top of what worked and was best for my body. How? Simple. Even as a kid I read everything I could get my hands on that taught me the best practices in nutrition and workouts.

But that wasn't enough. I took things a step further. When I was bodybuilding, everything I ate, every weight I pumped, even my naps, went into a journal. I hadn't journaled like that since I retired as a professional. But I got back into it when I started my 51-day journey to reclaim my ultimate body. Notice how close the words journey and journals are? With the success I had at age 48, I've made a commitment I'm going to keep journaling—because this is a journey that never ends!

That means that our homework never ends either, if we want to go to the next level. I'm a big believer in reading. I donate books to my kids' schools. As a businessman, I want to read what the best business authors are writing that can help me improve my company. I also continue to read cutting-edge books on health, nutrition, workouts, microbiotics, and anything else that can give me and my company an edge. I force myself to dig deep. If a book on microbiotics is more technical than I can understand as a nonscientist—I still push myself to learn as much as I can.

So what's the guaranteed way to get smarter—to improve your performance and practical knowledge? I know what you're thinking. It's obvious from what I've said above that the answer is reading. Well that's almost right, but there's something I want to add to that.

What happens when you read? You gain information, insights, and even inspiration from someone who has mastered a topic of interest to you. How can you not get smarter and sharper from reading people who know more than you? But that's where my bigger point comes in. The guaranteed way to get smarter is to surround yourself with smart people. That happens with books, periodicals, blogs, websites. And that also happens every day in real life interaction.

Am I smart enough to create the very best bodybuilding supplements in the world? Well, I feel I'm bright. I obviously have keen insights on what is needed. As someone who walks the walk, I have learned a lot through trial and error. But the answer is no. As gung-ho as I am to learn everything I possibly can, in order to be the best, I have to have smarter people working for me.

I'll never completely delegate research and development. Even if my team feels I'm in their way—I'm still going to be there. But I need team members with a high level of formal scientific education so they accomplish more than I ever could on my own. I make appearances and, believe me, I'm heavily involved in marketing my company. After all, my name is on it. But I still need the brightest and best marketing specialists I can find. If they want me to tweet, then fine, I'll utilize Instagram, Twitter and Facebook and everything else needed to spread the word. I need people who understand how all those things work together better than I ever can.

This 51-day journey really gave me a renewed shot of self-confidence. I feel that there is no limit to what I can do. I set a goal and accomplished it. In the same way, I believe there is no limit to what I can accomplish in business. The reason is simple: I'm smart enough to surround myself with the smartest people in the business!

The same holds true for you in every area of your life. Be true to your friends past and present whether you think they can do something for you or not. But never be intimidated by people who are smarter than you. In fact, seek them out and make them part of your world. Never stop learning. It's the guaranteed way for you to get smarter than ever before.

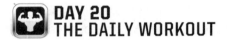

DAY 20
THE DAILY WORKOUT

THE MUSCLE BUILDER: REST

HARDGAINER WORKOUT: REST

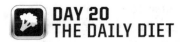

DAY 20
THE DAILY DIET

MEAL 1: Myofusion Shake: 2 scoops Myofusion, 1/2 cup egg whites, 2/3 cup instant oatmeal, 1 tablespoon natural peanut butter or almond butter, 1/2 cup apple juice, 1/2 cup water and ice.

MEAL 2: Myofusion Protein Pancakes: 1 scoop Myofusion, 1 cup egg whites, 1 cup oatmeal, 1/4 cup chopped walnuts, 1 sliced banana. Mix all together and cook on low heat on a non-stick pan using cooking spray. Optional: add sugar-free syrup.

MEAL 3: Same as Meal 1.

MEAL 4: 8 ounces lean buffalo patty *(or 93% lean ground beef)* with salsa or mustard, 1 cup brown rice, 6 ounces green salad with vinegar.

MEAL 5: 10 raw almonds.

MEAL 6: Egg Omelet: 1 cup egg whites mixed with 1 cup chopped peppers, onions, and tomatoes. 6 ounces green salad with vinegar and 1 slice watermelon on the side.

MEAL 7 *(optional)*: Same as Meal 1.

DAY 20 FOOD NOTE

My favorite fast meal is two scoops of Myofusion, four rice cakes, and a handful of almonds. I get my protein, complex carbohydrates, and essential fats.

DAY 20
THE DAILY TIP

You really need to eat seven times a day to keep your metabolism burning. That's hard. So realistically you will need to plan for some meal replacements. In a pinch, it's tough to beat a protein shake.

DAY 21 *EAT THAT FROG*

I read a little book once on personal development called *Eat That Frog* by Brian Tracy. What does eating the frog mean? To put it simply, every one of us has something important to get done today that we dread doing. It might not be as gross as eating a frog, but it's still distasteful to us. So we stall. We waste time. We get distracted easily. We move slowly. In other words, we procrastinate. The point of *Eat That Frog* was that instead of putting off what we hate to do, that is exactly what we should do first. Get it out of the way and move on. Our productivity will begin to soar.

When it comes to bodybuilding, most of us have a muscle group or body part that is most difficult for us to work on and that doesn't respond the way we expect. I could get big and rip my chest and arms just by looking at the weights. I may be exaggerating a bit, but building my chest and arms just weren't a problem for me. Abs, shoulders, back, glutes, upper legs—no problem. Lower legs? *Big* problem. My calf muscles just wouldn't respond for me like my other muscle groups.

What happens when we don't get the results we want? We get discouraged. We move on to something we like better. It's great that you can pump your arms up over eighteen inches without breaking a sweat, but if you have chicken legs, that's what needs improving. That's the frog that you have to eat.

I've put together a great daily schedule of exercises

and supersets for you. But if you have an area of your body that won't respond to your program, you need to switch the order and begin your workout with what needs the most attention first. What you least like to do. That's when your body has the most oxygen and fuel to focus on an area that is resistant to growth and development. In other words, eat the frog first!

If you were looking for a workout and nutrition program that was easy, you came to the wrong place. There are things I am asking you to do that you won't like. Building your best body ever is going to be tough work and mean eating some frogs. So hit what's hardest for you first. Don't mess around. Don't start chatting with everyone around you. Take it as a personal challenge. But here is the good news: frogs are high-protein and low-fat. So go for it!

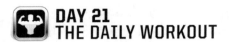

DAY 21
THE DAILY WORKOUT

THE MUSCLE BUILDER: REST

HARDGAINER WORKOUT: REST

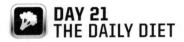

DAY 21
THE DAILY DIET

MEAL 1: Myofusion Shake: 2 scoops Myofusion, 1/2 cup egg whites, 2/3 cup instant oatmeal, 1 tablespoon natural peanut butter or almond butter, 1/2 cup apple juice, 1/2 cup water and ice.

MEAL 2: Myofusion Protein Pancakes: 1 scoop Myofusion, 1 cup egg whites, 1 cup oatmeal, 1/4 cup chopped walnuts, 1 sliced banana. Mix all together and cook on low heat on a non-stick pan using cooking spray. Optional: add sugar-free syrup.

MEAL 3: Same as Meal 1.

MEAL 4: 8 ounces grilled chicken breast, 1 cup brown rice, 1 cup steamed broccoli.

MEAL 5: Same as Meal 1.

MEAL 6: 8 ounces mahi mahi or other white fish, 1 small potato, 3 ounces steamed string beans, 4 ounces green salad with vinegar.

MEAL 7 *(optional)***:** Same as Meal 1.

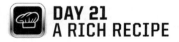

DAY 21
A RICH RECIPE

UNCLE SAM SMOOTHIE

2 tablespoons reduced-fat peanut butter

2 tablespoons flaxseed oil

2 - 3 scoops of Gaspari Nutrition delicious vanilla IsoFusion

16 ounces of water with ice

Combine all ingredients in a blender and blend until smooth. Pour into glasses and serve immediately. Makes 2 servings.

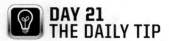

DAY 21
THE DAILY TIP

Quotes are a great way to get—and stay—inspired!

You may delay, but time will not.
–Benjamin Franklin

Only put off until tomorrow what you are willing to die having left undone.
–Pablo Picasso

You cannot escape the responsibility of tomorrow by evading it today.
–Abraham Lincoln

My advice I never do tomorrow what you can do today.
Procrastination is the thief of time.
–Charles Dickens

It is easier to resist at the beginning than at the end.
–Leonardo da Vinci

DAY 22 NO, IT WON'T KILL YOU!

Not long ago, I donated some money and equipment to my son's elementary school to give them a boost on getting certified for The President's Fitness Challenge. Originally established by President John F. Kennedy for school children, the President's Council of Fitness, Sports, and Nutrition has now expanded the scope of its mission to encourage people of all ages and abilities to become physically active and participate in sports. My friend Arnold Schwarzenegger served as Chair of the Council in the early 1990s. That may very well be how he got his start in politics.

I'm sure it comes as no surprise to you by now that I feel very strongly about the importance of living a healthy lifestyle, particularly one that includes plenty of physical activity. I believe that part of the solution to our nation's childhood obesity epidemic is getting our kids off the couch or away from their technological devices and teaching them the benefits and joys of exercise from a young age. More often than not, if a child has the opportunity to participate in sports, organized play, or fun physical activities, they not only feel better, but also develop a sense of accomplishment and pride in what they are doing.

So I was pleased to be able to support a program that would help both my kids and their friends learn to love exercise. You can imagine my surprise when my son came home one day and said, "Dad, all my friends are mad at you!"

Mad at me? I wondered. *What is this all about?*

I had a good laugh when he told me, "It's because all the stuff you gave the school means they have to work out so hard. You're killing us!"

Kids exaggerate—when they are hungry, they say they are "starving"—so I didn't make too big of a deal about what they said or try to over interpret it. But, really, their response wasn't all that different from what I hear every day from adults who don't really want to change their lives. It's easier to make excuses and not do anything about it.

I know too many men and women who are tired out and defeated before they even get out of the locker room and over to the weights. There's nothing wrong with them physically. They've simply bought into the crazy notion that hard work is bad. Or they simply can't do it. Or it surely will kill them.

You don't have to look very far or listen too closely to hear plenty of people who feel life is just way too hard. I know some people who work harder at complaining *about* what they need to do than actually *doing* it. It's pervasive in the workplace, in parenting, in health and nutrition. We've become a nation of whiners and "can't-do-its" instead of people who see endless possibilities and refuse to settle for less than the best life has to offer.

I'm going to say it over and over. Nothing worthwhile comes easy. I don't care if it's someone promising you easy money, easy weight loss, easy success. The old adage is true: if it sounds too good to be true, then it is. But just because something isn't easy doesn't mean it isn't possible. Or that it isn't worth it. Or that you shouldn't give everything you possibly can to make it a reality.

When you picked up this book and started the program, you made a decision to improve yourself. You knew I wasn't offering you an easy fix. What I am offering you is the joy and satisfaction of working hard and enjoying the fruits of your labor. Keep that positive attitude and momentum going.

I promise—it really won't kill you!

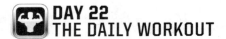

DAY 22
THE DAILY WORKOUT

THE MUSCLE BUILDER: CHEST & ABS
(Take 45 seconds - 1 minute rest between each set)
Incline dumbbell press – 4 sets of 8-10 reps
Incline dumbbell flies – 4 sets of 8-10 reps
Decline cable flies – 4 sets of 8-10 reps
Superset: Dumbbell flat bench, Pec Dec – 4 sets of 8-10 reps
Crunches – 4 sets of 25-30 reps
Leg raises – 4 sets of 25-30 reps

CARDIO
20-30 minutes interval cardio on treadmill

HARDGAINER WORKOUT: CHEST/BACK/BICEPS/TRICEPS/CORE
Modified Compound Superset #1 – *Take 45 seconds rest before moving on to the 2nd exercise*
Incline Dumbbell Press: 3 sets of 6-8 reps (45 Sec Rest)
Barbell Bent Over Row: 3 sets of 6-8 reps (1 min rest)
Modified Compound Superset #2 – *Take 45 seconds rest before moving on to the 2nd exercise*
Flat Dumbbell Bench Press: 3 sets of 6-8 reps (45 Sec Rest)
Chin-Ups: 3 sets of 6-8 reps (Strap on weight if you can)(1 min rest)
> *Note: If you cannot perform the Chin-up, either have someone spot you by using your legs off their hands for leverage or have them spot-push you up by the waist.*
Superset #3 – *No rest between exercises*
Barbell Curls: 3 sets of 8-10 reps (No Rest)
Close Grip Dumbbell Bench Press (Triceps): 3 sets of 8-10 reps (1 min rest)
Superset #4 – *No rest between exercises*
Dumbbell Hammer Curls: 3 sets of 10-12 reps (No Rest)
Triceps Pushdowns: 3 sets of 10-12 reps (1 min rest)
Superset #5 – *No rest between exercises*
Plank: 2 sets of 1 Minute Static Contraction (No Rest)
Bicycle Maneuver: 2 sets of 30 reps (1 min rest)

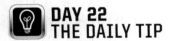

DAY 22
THE DAILY DIET

MEAL 1: Myofusion Shake: 2 scoops Myofusion, 1/2 cup egg whites, 2/3 cup instant oatmeal, 1 tablespoon natural peanut butter or almond butter, 1/2 cup apple juice, 1/2 cup water and ice.

MEAL 2: Myofusion Protein Pancakes: 1 scoop Myofusion, 1 cup egg whites, 1 cup oatmeal, 1/4 cup chopped walnuts, 1 sliced banana. Mix all together and cook on low heat on a non-stick pan using cooking spray. Optional: add sugar-free syrup.

MEAL 3: Same as Meal 1.

MEAL 4: Egg omelet: 1 cup egg whites mixed with 1 cup chopped peppers, onions, and tomatoes. 6 ounces green salad with vinegar, and 1 apple on the side.

MEAL 5: Same as Meal 1.

MEAL 6: 8 ounces of lean steak, 1 sweet potato, 1 cup raw kale salad with 1 teaspoon olive oil and lemon juice.

MEAL 7*[optional]***:** Same as Meal 1.

DAY 22
THE DAILY TIP

You have to think and feel positive to do your best. "That which doesn't kill us makes us stronger."

DAY 23 IT'S ALL ABOUT YOU

When I first started in bodybuilding, it was a small niche community. But what it lacked in numbers was more than made up for in commitment and intensity. As is the case now, there was a near-rabid cult following, and the center of the bodybuilding universe was located in Venice Beach in California.

When I first became a professional, the sport was taking off. Nothing brought awareness to hard core muscle-ripping bodybuilding than the documentary *Pumping Iron* that featured a relatively unknown athlete from Austria with a name that no one knew how to pronounce. People quickly learned how to say Arnold's last name as he skyrocketed to fame and fortune as an actor, later going on to serve as governor of California. In bodybuilding circles, we would say that Arnold got bigger as he got smaller.

But it wasn't just Arnold Schwarzenegger. Lou Ferrigno, Lee Haney, Franco Columbo, and other bodybuilders that followed Arnold became as close to household names as you could without being a musician, actor, or pro basketball player.

I think I was part of that growth. I did almost 80 magazine covers over a decade. Not everyone knew my name, but if someone ever had to wait in a checkout line at a supermarket or convenience store, they knew my smiling face and my body—even if they looked at the female model first when I shared the cover!

Bodybuilding probably peaked in popularity and participation in the 90s. It remains strong and continues to grow as a whole, but the form of bodybuilding I participated in—getting as big and ripped as possible—is staying about the same. Does that discourage me? Does that make me worry about the future of my company?

Not in the least!

And the reason is great news for all of us. People are into physical fitness like never before. Men and women, young and old, are heading to the gym, buying exercise equipment, learning about nutrition, and attempting to create a more positive lifestyle and healthy body for themselves. Bodybuilding will always have a presence and there are still plenty of diehard fans along with participants who are going to push their muscularity and physiques to the limits.

If you don't believe me, visit The Arnold Classic in Columbus, Ohio. It's held in early March every year. It used to be all about bodybuilding. Now there is a major MMA card, boxing, the Ohio high school wrestling tournament, judo, gymnastics, powerlifting, and tons of other competitions that showcase physical achievement. Visit the exhibition center where hundreds of booths feature the latest in sports equipment, apparel, and nutrition, as companies like mine introduce new information and products.

But the fitness craze isn't going anywhere. You've seen it. There is every kind of training center imaginable now. You even see 24/7 fitness clubs in strip malls. People are more into taking care of their bodies with the right exercise, diet, and supplements. Teachers, lawyers, doctors, insurance salespersons, housewives, factory workers, young teens, senior adults—there's no boundaries. And if you looked at this from a purely business standpoint, there's a whole lot more people out there who need to join the craze. The supply of new customers seems unlimited.

So bodybuilding has changed. The hardcore bodybuilding is there, but like when I started, it's more of a niche crowd. But overall, fitness has grown—and to me, that's what matters most.

Which brings up the subject of you. *51 Days: No Excuses* is not about Rich Gaspari. It's about you. It's not about my goals. It's about your goals.

Earlier I asked you to cut out a picture that showed the kind of body you wanted to build through this program. I asked you to do that so you would have a visual reminder of what you wanted to accomplish. Take a look at that picture again. Are you sure it's what you want? If so, go for it. If this program and learning more about yourself has led you to rethink exactly what you want to accomplish—it's no problem at all. Adjust your thinking appropriately—as long as you aren't quitting on what you really want.

Why? It's all about you.

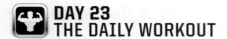

DAY 23
THE DAILY WORKOUT

THE MUSCLE BUILDER: BACK & CALVES
(Take 45 seconds - 1 minute rest between each set)
Deadlifts – 4 sets of 8-10 reps
Wide grip chins – 4 sets of 8-10 reps
Superset: Close grip pulldowns, Wide grip cable pullovers – 4 sets
of 8-10 reps
Superset: Cable low rows, T-bar rows – 4 sets of 8-10 reps
Superset: Two arm dumbbell rows, machine rows – 4 sets of 8-10 reps
Standing Calf raises – 5 sets of 15 reps
Seated calf raises – 5 sets of 15 reps

CARDIO
20-30 minutes interval cardio on treadmill

HARDGAINER WORKOUT:
THIGHS/HAMSTRINGS/DELTS/CALVES/LOWER ABS
Superset #1
Wide Stance Squats: 3 sets of 8-10 reps (45 Seconds Rest)
Stiff Legged Barbell Deadlifts: 3 sets of 8-10 reps (1 min rest)

> *Note: Utilize the "Full Body Tension Technique". This is when you
> stay in proper anatomical form and maintain that posture by
> keeping all of your major muscles contracted before & throughout
> the movements—this will keep you safe, while allowing you to use
> maximum intensity.*

Giant Set #2 – *3 exercises performed back-to-back without rest*
Leg Press: 3 sets of 6-8 reps (No Rest)
Leg Extensions: 3 sets of 10-12 reps (No Rest)
Lying Leg Curls: 3 sets of 10-12 reps (1 min rest)
Giant Set #3
Upright Barbell Row: 3 sets of 8-10 reps (No Rest)
Lateral Raises: 3 sets of 8-10 reps (No Rest)
Descending Set #4 – *Drop the weight as you move from set–to-set*

Standing Calf Raises (Gastrocs) - 3 Descending Sets – Decrease
weight as you descend, if necessary:
- 1st set of 12-15 reps (15 sec rest)
- 2nd set of 12-15 reps (15 sec rest)
- 3rd set of 12-15 reps (1 min rest & repeat 2 more times)

Superset #5

Bent Over Lateral Dumbbell Raises: 3 sets of 10-12 reps (No Rest)

Seated Calf Raises (Soleus): 3 sets of 10-12 reps (1 min rest)

Hanging Leg Raises: 3 sets of 15-20 reps (1 min rest)

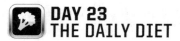 **DAY 23**
THE DAILY DIET

MEAL 1: Myofusion Shake: 2 scoops Myofusion, 1/2 cup egg whites, 2/3 cup instant oatmeal, 1 tablespoon natural peanut butter or almond butter, 1/2 cup apple juice, 1/2 cup water and ice.

MEAL 2: Myofusion Protein Pancakes: 1 scoop Myofusion, 1 cup egg whites, 1 cup oatmeal, 1/4 cup chopped walnuts, 1 sliced banana. Mix all together and cook on low heat on a non-stick pan using cooking spray. Optional: add sugar-free syrup.

MEAL 3: Same as Meal 1.

MEAL 4: 8 ounces grilled tuna, 1 cup brown rice, 1 teaspoon of olive oil, 1 cup steamed green beans.

MEAL 5: 10 raw almonds.

MEAL 6: 8 ounces lean ground beef, 1 cup gluten-free pasta, 4-6 ounces low sodium natural tomato sauce with 1 tablespoon grated cheese (optional).

MEAL 7 (optional): Same as Meal 1.

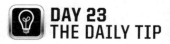 **DAY 23**
THE DAILY TIP

Deadlifts are great for the back and other body parts. Work with lighter weights until you build strength and have the correct form perfected. Ultimately, your own body weight should be the measure you use.

DAY 24 NOT FUN AND GAMES

I love hitting the road and meeting with fans and customers all over the world. One of the comments I often hear in my travels is, "You look great Rich—not like you use to look, but still great."

Having lived in the world of bodybuilding so long I am used to getting kidded with. When I did my first nude photograph—and I would quickly add that it was a tasteful, modest, discreet profile pose—my family and friends really gave me the business. I thought it was great. If you can't laugh along with others—even if you are laughing at yourself at the time—then you are taking things way too seriously. Make time to lighten up and laugh. It's good for you emotionally and physically.

But there are also times when you don't joke around. For me, that was in the gym. I'm not going to try and tell people how to conduct themselves during a workout. I know there are different personality types. I am a little more private and focused. Others need to talk and chat almost as much as they need to eat and breathe. But I am still going to stress that if you are going to build your ultimate body, workout time needs to be intense and focused. Two individuals can read this book and do the same exercises. One feels like a puddle of Jell-O when he is done. The other talks a great game but really doesn't push it hard. He doesn't work his muscles close to the point of exhaustion. Who do you think is going to have the best results?

It usually comes down to a lack of focus. And a lack of focus is usually a matter of wanting workout time to be about fun and games. I want you to have a great time. I want you to stay motivated and look forward to pushing yourself. But I can't make it fun all the time.

When I hit the gym, it is all business. That's the reason that Lee Haney, Hulk Hogan, Steve Borden (Sting), Arnold Schwarzenegger, and others wanted to work out with me. They knew that they would be pushing themselves harder than at any other time. They knew they were going to get a lot done. They also knew they were going to be hurting when the workout was over.

I want you to push yourself so hard you don't have the breath to chat or tell a joke. I don't want you pacing yourself. I want you to squeeze every last ounce of energy you have. I want you to make those muscles burn. Don't save yourself for anything else.

After today? Same thing tomorrow. Doesn't that sound like fun? There's plenty of time to laugh and tell jokes. But I guarantee when you see how your body responds to a serious, intense, focused workout, the smile on your face will last a whole lot longer than the latest joke.

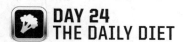

DAY 24
THE DAILY WORKOUT

THE MUSCLE BUILDER: LEGS
(Take 45 seconds - 1 minute rest between each set)
Lying leg curls – 5 sets of 10-12 reps
Stiff-legged deadlifts – 4 sets of 10-12 reps
Leg extensions – 5 sets of 10-12 reps (double drop set on last set)
45-degree Leg Press – 4 sets of 15 reps (double drop set on last set)
Hack Squat – 3 sets of 15 reps (triple drop set on last set)
Superset: Squats, walking lunges – 3 sets of 15-20 reps

CARDIO
20-30 minutes interval cardio on treadmill

HARDGAINER WORKOUT: REST

DAY 24
THE DAILY DIET

MEAL 1: Myofusion Shake: 2 scoops Myofusion, 1/2 cup egg whites, 2/3 cup instant oatmeal, 1 tablespoon natural peanut butter or almond butter, 1/2 cup apple juice, 1/2 cup water and ice.
MEAL 2: Myofusion Protein Pancakes: 1 scoop Myofusion, 1 cup egg whites, 1 cup oatmeal, 1/4 cup chopped walnuts, 1 sliced banana. Mix all together and cook on low heat on a non-stick pan using cooking spray. Optional: add sugar-free syrup.
MEAL 3: 10 raw almonds.
MEAL 4: 8 ounces grilled chicken, 1 cup brown rice, 1 tablespoon olive oil or salad dressing with 1 cup veggies.
MEAL 5: Same as meal 1.
MEAL 6: 8 ounces lean buffalo patty *(or 93% lean ground beef)* with salsa or mustard, 1 small potato, 1 cup raw kale salad with 1 teaspoon olive oil and lemon juice.
MEAL 7 *(optional)*: Same as Meal 1.

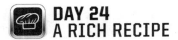

DAY 24
A RICH RECIPE

RAW KALE SALAD WITH LEMON AND PARMESAN

 1/4 cup lemon juice

 1/2 cup olive oil

 1 bunch kale

 1/2 cup pine nuts or sliced almonds

 1/4 cup shredded parmesan cheese

 2 tablespoons fresh lemon zest, (optional)

 sea salt and pepper, to taste

Wash and dry the kale. Remove the stems and chop it into thin strips by rolling the leaves into a ball and making thin slices.

In a small bowl, thoroughly whisk together the lemon juice and olive oil. Add the nuts and parmesan to the greens and toss to combine. Drizzle the dressing over the greens, and toss to combine. Sprinkle salad with lemon zest to garnish and top with sea salt and cracked pepper to taste. Makes 8 servings.

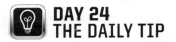

DAY 24
THE DAILY TIP

Eating on the road is tough, but not impossible. But now, even fast food restaurants have grilled chicken and salads. However, be mindful of sauces and dressings to make sure you stay on track.

DAY 25 "YOU CAN'T DO THAT" AND OTHER MOTIVATIONAL SPEECHES

Growing up I always knew I was loved and that my family had my back. That was a great feeling then and also later in life when things weren't going so great for me. I can't thank my parents enough. But just because my dad loved me doesn't mean he was always easy to be around. He had his own bodybuilding program planned for me. It was called hard work in the trenches as a manual laborer. He was a brick and stonemason, so he certainly knew a fail proof system to get me strong. Now, I'm proud of my dad and don't think of myself as being above manual labor—that's just not what I wanted. I was mesmerized by the world of bodybuilding.

When I first showed my dad the pictures of Lou, Arnold, Franco, Samir, and others to explain why I was eating a dozen eggs and drinking a whole gallon of milk each day, his immediate response was "you can't do that." When he found out I was sneaking into the weight room at Rutgers University, all he said to me was "you can't do that." When I left Rutgers before graduating to pursue my dream of being a bodybuilder in California, the capital of the bodybuilding world, once again he said to me, "you can't do that."

The problem for my dad was that he raised me to be independent, to take chances—and to work hard. So his words didn't discourage me and obviously I didn't agree with his opinion. I can honestly say that him telling me, "you can't do it" was a great motivator. I wasn't mad. I wasn't trying to get back at him. But I did want to prove him wrong. I wanted him to be proud of me. And I succeeded in that endeavor.

When I turned professional and writers and other competitors said I couldn't become a champion because I was too small, I have to admit part of my motivation was to prove them wrong. I never wasted much emotional energy on it, but I'd be lying if I said I didn't get any satisfaction from hearing people who said I couldn't succeed, have to explain how I did it.

Motivation can come from a number of different directions. Most importantly and best of all is when it is internal and tied to your own dreams and goals. But we all need the extra boost of motivation we get once in a while from an encouraging word from a coach, a boss, a parent, a friend, or a competitor. I'm sure you can think of someone who has had that kind of impact in your life. Don't forget to return the favor and encourage others.

The good news is we can also turn any negativity that comes our way into a motivational tool. I grew up when dads let the belt do their talking. Fear of punishment definitely motivated me. A rebuke, a bad performance review at work, a low grade on a test, someone mouthing off to you—so-called experts today shudder at the very thought of such negative confrontations. They are terrified it's going to ruin your self-esteem and short circuit healthy development. And too many people believe the experts and settle for mediocrity rather than challenge someone to do better.

I'm not going to tell you that you can't build your ultimate body, because I know you can. But I kind of hope someone else does. And I hope it gets you mad or frustrated or whatever other emotion you need to harness to get yourself motivated and determined to succeed. The next time someone tells you that you don't have what it takes, tell that person, "Thank you." Then go out and prove them wrong.

DAY 25
THE DAILY WORKOUT

THE MUSCLE BUILDER: SHOULDERS & ABS
(Take 45 seconds - 1 minute rest between each set)
Seated barbell front press – 4 sets of 8-12 reps
Giantset: Seated side laterals, Arnold Press, Standing dumbbell upright rows – 4 sets of 10-12 reps
Incline one arm side laterals – 3 sets of 12-15
Machine rear laterals – 4 sets of 12-15
Barbell shrugs from behind – 4 sets of 12-15
Twisting crunches – 4 sets of 30 reps
Leg raises – 4 sets of 25 reps

CARDIO
20-30 minutes interval cardio on treadmill

HARDGAINER WORKOUT: CHEST/BACK/BICEPS/TRICEPS/ABS
Modified Compound Superset #1
Flat Dumbbell Bench Press: 3 sets of 8, 6, 4 reps [90 second rest]
Close Grip Neutral Grip Pull-Ups: 3 sets of 8, 6, 4 reps
[Strap weight on if you can – 2 mins rest]
Note: If you cannot perform the Close Grip Pull-Up, either have someone spot you by using your legs off their hands for leverage or have them spot-push you up by the waist.
Modified Compound Superset #2
Incline Barbell Bench Press: 3 sets of 8, 6, 4 reps [90 second rest]
Bent Over Underhand Barbell Row: 3 sets of 8, 6, 4 reps [2 min rest]
Giant Modified Compound Super Set #3 – *Take prescribed rest between exercise*
Chest Dips: 3 sets of 8, 6, 4 reps [60 second rest]
Preacher Curls: 3 sets of 8, 6, 4 reps [45 second rest]
Close Grip Bench Press: 3 sets of 8, 6, 4 reps [2 min rest]
Giant Modified Compound Super Set #4
E-Z Preacher Curls: 3 sets of 8, 6, 4 reps [60 second rest]
Lying Triceps Extensions: 3 sets of 8, 6, 4 reps [45 second rest]

Swiss Ball (aka "Inflated Fitness Ball") Crunches: 3 sets of 20, 15, 10 reps (Hold a weight plate or dumbbell overhead if you can) (2 min rest)

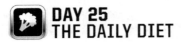

DAY 25
THE DAILY DIET

MEAL 1: Myofusion Shake: 2 scoops Myofusion, 1/2 cup egg whites, 2/3 cup instant oatmeal, 1 tablespoon natural peanut butter or almond butter, 1/2 cup apple juice, 1/2 cup water and ice.

MEAL 2: Myofusion Protein Pancakes: 1 scoop Myofusion, 1 cup egg whites, 1 cup oatmeal, 1/4 cup chopped walnuts, 1 sliced banana. Mix all together and cook on low heat on a non-stick pan using cooking spray. Optional: add sugar-free syrup.

MEAL 3: Same as Meal 1.

MEAL 4: Egg omelet: 1cup egg whites mixed with 1 cup chopped peppers, onions, and tomatoes. 6 ounces green salad with vinegar and 1 apple on the side.

MEAL 5: Same as Meal 1.

MEAL 6: 8 ounces baked salmon, 1 cup quinoa, 1 cup asparagus.

MEAL 7 *(optional)*: Same as Meal 1.

DAY 25
THE DAILY TIP

Are you passionate about cycling? All good cyclists are able to break away, climb hills with endurance, and sprint at the end of race. The aim is to make your body healthy enough to accomplish recovery and tissue repair. Plus, you must maintain a high strength-to-weight ratio. The following supplement guidelines can help you achieve your goals:

- **Pre-season and Season Recommended Supplements:** multivitamins, multiminerals, antioxidants, fatty acids, branched-chain amino acids, low-calorie protein drink, carbohydrate drinks, fat-burning supplements, anabolics.
- **Pre-race Recommended Supplements:** branched-chain amino acids, low-calorie protein drink, carbohydrate drinks.

DAY 26 NOTHING WORTHWHILE IS EASY

When I was a professional bodybuilder, I only made a little from the competitions and a few extra bucks from endorsements. But it wasn't a sport that was going to make me rich. Although the health and fitness boom had begun, it didn't have the pervasive market presence it does today. And bodybuilding was a pretty small slice of the pie.

That's one of the reasons I love sponsoring athletes. We have both amateurs and professionals in our lineup of featured athletes. What do they do for us? A lot! This is going to come as no surprise to you, but my philosophy of working with athletes is a little different than that of other companies—and it is based on what my dad taught me as a kid: it's all about your work ethic.

I want our athletes to do well financially. I don't want them wondering whether they are doing the right thing in pursuing their passion because they always have to worry about finances like my generation of bodybuilders did. I want them to be successful now and also help set them up for a smoother transition to life after competition than I had. But I want them learn the value of hard work. And that means I only hire workers.

At times I've had agents and athletes approach me to become part of Team Gaspari and I have had to say no. Not because they aren't talented and successful. They don't want to work like my team does. A lot of companies give contracts and write checks to bodybuilders and other athletes with pretty low expectations. Maybe they do a formal photo shoot or two and then make three appearances per year to say they use their product.

We pay better than most—but we also make our athletes work. Three or four appearances per year? We require four or five per month instead. Making appearances isn't just about showing up with a smile on your face. You have to be in top shape and you have to work hard to get pumped up before you ever stand in front of a microphone and camera. I've heard some competitors who want us to sponsor them say, "That's a lot of work!" I tell them most of us have to work at least five days a week. My dad laid brick and stone five or six days a week. Now *that's* real work!

We're not just about appearances, we want athletes who are active in their sport. We want competitors. One of the toughest jobs in my company is effectively managing our athletes' appearance schedules around competitions and the hardcore, focused training schedules that lead up to any event. We also want them to pass along their knowledge, so we help them with blogs and video blogs.

The reward we get is obvious: positive publicity for Gaspari Nutrition. What do they get? A nice supplemental income that allows them to commit wholeheartedly to their sport and at the same time, the opportunity to build their own brand. We really do want our team members to be more successful competitively, financially, and in fame than they ever could on their own. I'm glad for all the sacrifices I made and would do it all again. They make sacrifices, too. I just want it to be better for them than it was for me.

I have a real simple point in all this: nothing worthwhile in life is easy. I guess you might win the lottery—but how many lottery winners do you know who find themselves in much better circumstances after they get the fast cash? The numbers are pretty shocking—the vast majority simply can't handle all that "easy money," and they usually lose it all—sometimes finding themselves in worse straits then before. They think they can get rich without working hard for it, and will then have the discipline and understanding to manage all that wealth. No, life doesn't work that way.

If you looked at the title of this book and thought I was offering you something easy, I apologize. I am confident you can accomplish some incredible things in 51 days. But, I never want to imply that this is easy.

But I've got a nice reward I'm offering you—your best body ever. But you have to work for it! Nothing worthwhile is easy.

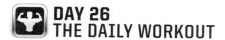 DAY 26
THE DAILY WORKOUT

THE MUSCLE BUILDER: BICEPS & TRICEPS
[Take 45 seconds - 1 minute rest between each set]

Superset: Incline dumbbell curls, Rope pushdowns – 4 sets of 10 reps

Superset: Standing barbell curls, Seated 2-arm overhead tricep extension with Dumbbell – 4 sets of 10 reps

Superset: Seated preacher curls with EZ curl bar, Lying pullover press – 4 sets of 10 reps

Superset: Dumbbell concentration curls, cable kickbacks – 4 sets of 10 reps

CARDIO
20-30 minutes interval cardio on treadmill

HARDGAINER WORKOUT: THIGHS/HAMSTRINGS/DELTS/CALVES
Modified Compound Superset #1

Medium Stance Squats: 3 sets of 8, 6, 4 reps (90 second rest)

Lying Leg Curls: 3 sets of 8, 6, 4 reps (90 second rest)

> *Note: If you suffer from lower back problems you may substitute the squat for the leg press. Since you are performing the leg press as your second exercise, then just use a close stance on this one and a medium stance on the second one.*

Modified Compound Superset #2

Leg Press: 3 sets of 8, 6, 4 reps (90 second rest)

Barbell Romanian Deadlifts: 3 sets of 8, 6, 4 reps (2 min rest)

Modified Compound Superset #3

Seated Barbell Front Shoulder: 3 sets of 8, 6, 4 reps (60 second rest)

Standing Calf Raise (Gastrocs): 3 sets of 10, 8, 6 reps (2 min rest)

Modified Compound Superset #4

Dumbbell Lateral Raises: 3 sets of 8, 6, 4 reps (60 second rest)

Lying Leg Raises with a pop at the top of each rep: 3 sets of 10, 8, 6 reps (60 second rest)

Descending Set #5 – *Drop the weight as you move from set-to-set*

Seated Calf Raises (Soleus) - 3 Descending Sets – *Decrease weight as you descend, if necessary*
- 1st set of 12-15 reps (15 sec rest)
- 2nd set of 12-15 reps (15 sec rest)
- 3rd set of 12-15 reps (1 min rest & repeat 2 more times)

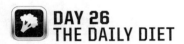

DAY 26
THE DAILY DIET

MEAL 1: Myofusion Shake: 2 scoops Myofusion, 1/2 cup egg whites, 2/3 cup instant oatmeal, 1 tablespoon natural peanut butter or almond butter, 1/2 cup apple juice, 1/2 cup water and ice.

MEAL 2: Myofusion Protein Pancakes: 1 scoop Myofusion, 1 cup egg whites, 1 cup oatmeal, 1/4 cup chopped walnuts, 1 sliced banana. Mix all together and cook on low heat on a non-stick pan using cooking spray. Optional: add sugar-free syrup.

MEAL 3: Same as Meal 1.

MEAL 4: 8 ounces grilled chicken, 1 cup brown rice, 1 tablespoon olive oil or salad dressing with 1 cup veggies.

MEAL 5: 10 raw almonds.

MEAL 6: 8 ounces of lean steak, 1 sweet potato, 1 cup raw kale salad with 1 teaspoon olive oil and lemon juice.

MEAL 7 [optional]**:** Same as Meal 1.

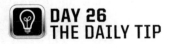

DAY 26
THE DAILY TIP

To get big arms you have to have great triceps. I like to start with the tricep pushdown with a rope or v-bar. This really isolates the muscle. Make sure you feel the burn in your triceps so you aren't getting help from other muscles.

DAY 27 AGING WITH STYLE

What are the keys to aging gracefully? I'm no expert on the subject but I've read enough to know that the usual suspects are:

- How you handle stress
- Your attitude—are you positive or negative?
- Your mental activity
- Your physical activity
- Your diet
- Rest and sleep

Even if genetics is the biggest factor in how we age, the above list gives us plenty to work on that's under our control.

You are almost a full month into training with me. I'd like you to look at the list above and think about what you've being doing.

Oh, by the way, if you're a young pup that isn't sure why I even bring this up, just remember I've been where you are—but are you going to be able to be where I am when you're 48? What you do today will have a huge impact on what you are able to do 10 years from now.

Back to the list. This book isn't specifically about handling stress, but psychologists and physiologists will tell you that rigorous physical activity is a tremendous stress reliever. Check that one off.

This book, by design, is all about a positive attitude. I've asked you to make goals, to believe in yourself, to fight through adversity and disappointment, to hang with people that motivate you, and a whole lot more. If you make the total program in this book—including the attitude I espouse—don't you think you will be creating the best mental outlook for aging gracefully?

I've challenged you to study and to be a lifelong learner, but I'm not going to make any claims that this book outlines a program to keep you mentally sharp—though again, physiologists will tell you that if you let your body go to seed, your mental acuity will be negatively impacted. But I'm leaving it up to you to do your crosswords and Sudoku and read books and take classes to keep your brain "muscle" stimulated.

When you look up at the last three items on the list, physical activity, diet, and rest, I've bombarded you with how important each discipline is to reaching your goal of achieving your ultimate body. Big but lean; strong; ripped. If you've missed those three points then you haven't been reading or you're in such a hurry you haven't paid attention.

Guess what? Those same disciplines you are doing as part of your march to your ultimate body are what will keep you youthful at every age in the life span.

When I embarked on this crazy 51-day quest, I was told countless times that there was no way I could get into competition form. Why? *You're too old Rich. You're almost 50. It's a young man's sport.*

Thank God I hadn't let myself go so I had a base to work from. But I'm also thankful I was challenged to think and act young. I like what I got done at 48 but I firmly believe it will pay dividends when I'm 58.

One of the men I most admire is Jack LeLanne. He is known as the "godfather of fitness." He died in 2011 at the age of 96. After he beat 21-year-old Arnold Schwarzenegger in an informal bodybuilding contest at age 54, Arnold simply said, "That Jack LaLanne is an animal." He preached fitness and diet until his death—and he continued to accomplish incredible acts of strength in his 90s.

When you think about aging with style, take Jack's words to heart that he spoke shortly before he died: *"I train like I'm training for the Olympics or for a Mr. America contest, the way I've always trained my whole life. You see, life is a battlefield. Life is survival of the fittest. How many healthy people do you know? How many happy people do you know? Think about it. People work at dying, they don't work at living. My workout is my obligation to life. It's my tranquilizer. It's part of the way I tell the truth — and telling the truth is what's kept me going all these years."*

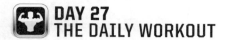

DAY 27
THE DAILY WORKOUT

THE MUSCLE BUILDER: REST

HARDGAINER WORKOUT: REST

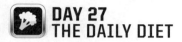

DAY 27
THE DAILY DIET

MEAL 1: Myofusion Shake: 2 scoops Myofusion, 1/2 cup egg whites, 2/3 cup instant oatmeal, 1 tablespoon natural peanut butter or almond butter, 1/2 cup apple juice, 1/2 cup water and ice.

MEAL 2: Myofusion Protein Pancakes: 1 scoop Myofusion, 1 cup egg whites, 1 cup oatmeal, 1/4 cup chopped walnuts, 1 sliced banana. Mix all together and cook on low heat on a non-stick pan using cooking spray. Optional: add sugar-free syrup.

MEAL 3: Same as Meal 1.

MEAL 4: 8 ounces grilled chicken mixed with 1 cup brown rice, 1 tablespoon olive oil or salad dressing with 1 cup veggies.

MEAL 5: Same as Meal 1.

MEAL 6: 8 ounces lean ground beef, 1 cup gluten-free pasta, 4-6 ounces low sodium natural tomato sauce with 1 tablespoon grated cheese *[optional]*.

MEAL 7 *[optional]*: Same as Meal 1.

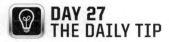

DAY 27
THE DAILY TIP

It takes a lot of dedication to build your ultimate body. You still need stay well rounded socially, emotionally, and mentally. On rest days, make sure you schedule some friendship time.

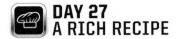 **DAY 27**
A RICH RECIPE

DUTCH CHOCO-NUT ICE CREAM

1 cup skim milk

1 cup milk

2 - 3 scoops of Gaspari Nutrition Milk Chocolate IsoFusion

2 egg whites

1 teaspoon vanilla extract

zero-calorie sweetener, such as Stevia, to taste

1/3 cup chopped hazelnuts

Put the egg whites in boiling water for 30 seconds just to lightly poach them. Remove the egg whites from the water and put them in a blender. Add the skim milk, milk, sweetener, vanilla extract, and Gaspari Nutrition Milk Chocolate Isofusion and blend until smooth. Add the chopped hazelnuts, blend again. Pour into serving glasses, and refrigerate until ready to eat. Makes 4 servings.

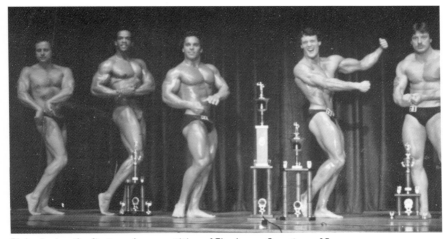

Rich winning the first men's competition of The Jersey Cup at age 19.

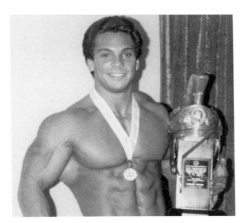

Rich proudly displaying his Mr. Universe trophy (1984).

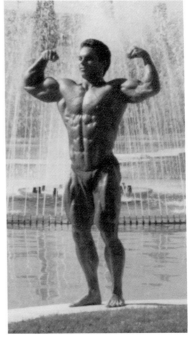

Rich at Caesar's Palace, Las Vegas, after winning the Mr. Universe competition (1984).

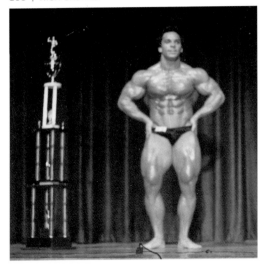

Rich posing beside his trophy at The Jersey Cup (1983).

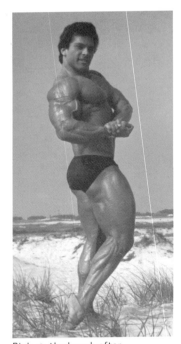

Rich on the beach after The Junior Nationals (1983).

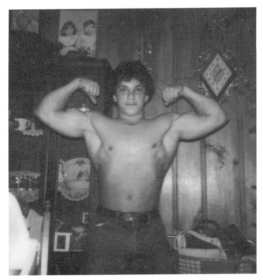

15-year-old Rich at home in New Jersey after training for one year.

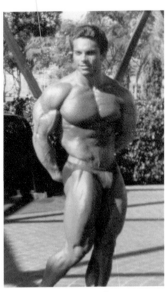

Rich in New Orleans after winning the 1984 Nationals.

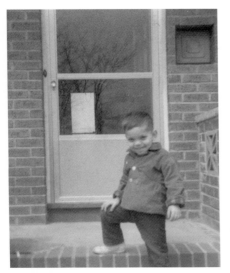

Rich at age 3 with that fierce, determined look!

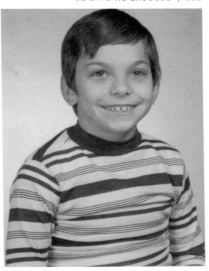

Rich's school yearbook photo at age 11.

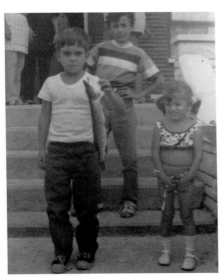

The first fish Rich ever caught (age 11).

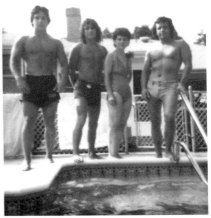

Rich at home in Edison, New Jersey, with his brothers Gaetano and Michael, and sister Zena.

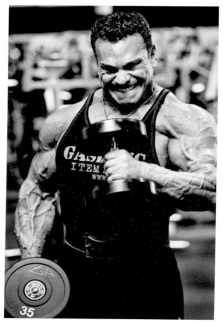

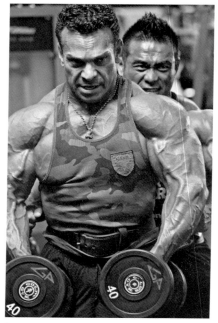

Rich doing a curl after his transformation.
Photo courtesy of Per Bernal.

Rich doing a side a lateral with
Hidetada Yamagishi.
Photo courtesy of Per Bernal.

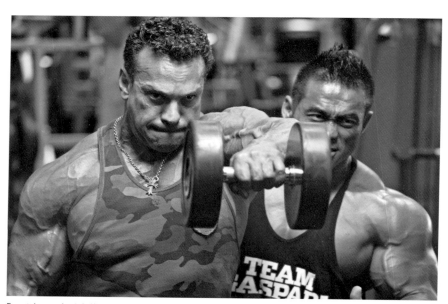

Front lateral with Hidetada Yamagishi after his transformation.
Photo courtesy of Per Bernal.

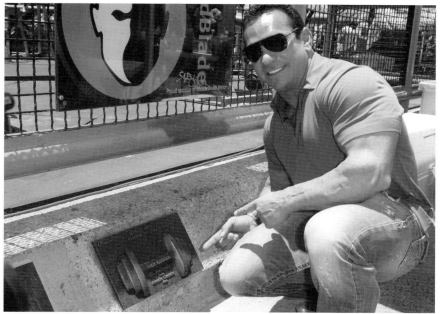

2011 Muscle Beach Walk of Fame plaque.

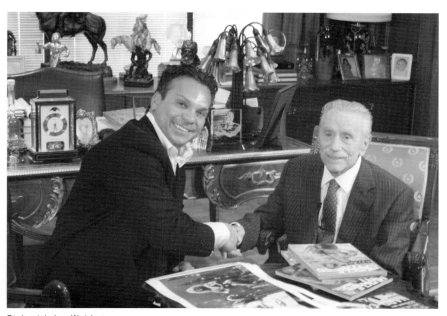

Rich with Joe Weider.

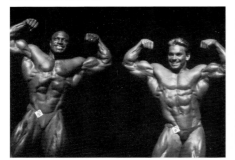

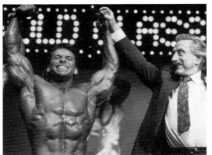

Rich with Lee Haney at the 1988
Mr. Olympia receiving 2nd place.

Rich, with Joe Weider, after winning the
first Arnold Classic in 1989.

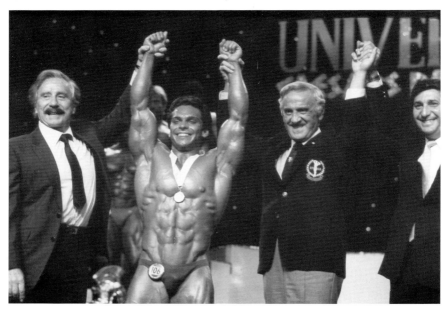

1984 Mr. Universe competition at Caesar's Palace. Rich with Joe and Ben Weider.

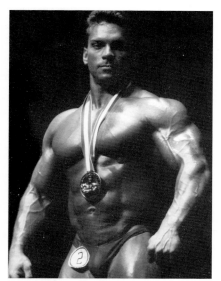

Rich proudly displaying his medal at Mr. Olympia in 1986.

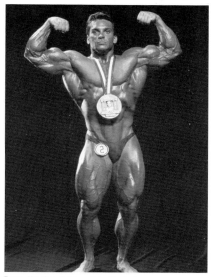

Proudly displaying his 2nd place Mr. Olympia medal in 1986.

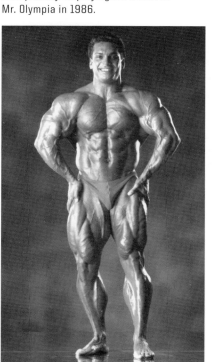

Candid pose in 1987. Photo courtesy of Mike Neveau.

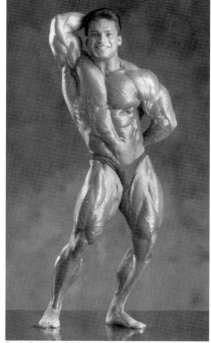

Rich Posing. 1988. Photo courtesy of Mike Neveau.

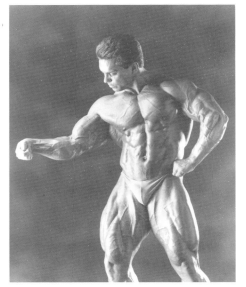

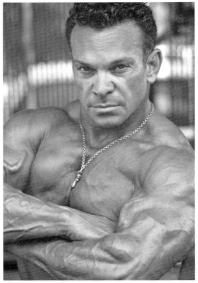

Rich Posing. 1986. Photo courtesy of Chris Lund.

Rich doing his serious pose after his transformation in 2011.
Photo courtesy of Per Bernal.

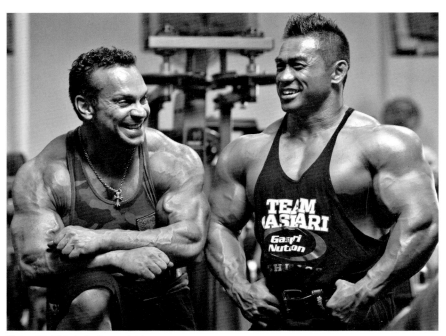

Rich with Hidetada Yamagishi. Photo courtesy of Per Bernal.

DAY 28 WHO WAS THE GREATEST?

The first "Super Bowl" of Professional Bodybuilding was held on September 18, 1965, at the Brooklyn Academy of Music in New York City. In an effort to enable Mr. Universe winners to continue competing and earn money, Joe Weider founded Mr. Olympia as bodybuilding's first professional event.

I don't know if the event made the man or the man made the event, but the first Mr. Olympia champion was Larry Scott, who would go on to repeat the following year. Larry was the first bodybuilding superstar—he brought a size and shape that had not been seen before. But more importantly, his unique aura, personality, and charisma helped launch a new professional sport.

As I write this book, the elite Mr. Olympia "club" has only thirteen members. Chris Dickerson (1982), Sammir Bannout (1983), and Dexter Jackson (2008), are the only three who haven't won multiple titles. Phil Heath unseated the massive Jay Cutler.

Just five years after Larry Scott's first win, Arnold Schwarzenegger changed the sport yet again—and even more dramatically than Larry had. He had perfect symmetry and an incredible shape that flowed both directions from a tiny waist. He was intense and charismatic in his own unique way, and he would go on to win seven titles between 1970 and 1980.

A lot of the people think the 80s were the most competitive era of professional bodybuilding. Lee Haney set new standards of size and shape combined with shredding on his way to eight straight victories. I pushed him as hard as I could. I thought maybe I had him in 1988. I had support on that from a number of experts. But bottom line, his combination of ripped muscle and size were incredible—and to knock off the champion you have to do it decisively.

Maybe the only bodybuilder who was more natural—because it is well documented he didn't have to diet and work at the same level as mere mortals like me—was Sergio Olivo. He owned the title for the three years before the Arnold era. In my opinion, Sergio and Lee were perhaps the two most genetically gifted bodybuilders of all time.

I didn't think anyone could approach Haney for wins, but then there was Dorian Yates, who won six straight before retiring. But that was just a warm-up for the next great champion, Ronnie Coleman, who did match Lee's eight straight victories. What more can I say? As technology, supplementation, and overall knowledge grew, so did the champions. Each decade saw dramatic jumps in both size and definition of ripped muscle. Coleman was competing at 270 pounds with the definition you would never have seen on a bodybuilder with that much size twenty years earlier. So it was no surprise when Jay Cutler competed and won four titles at 290 pounds.

So many great competitors, so many undeniable champions. But who was best? In other words, who was the greatest bodybuilder of all time? As any sports fan knows it's tough to compare players from different eras. Babe Ruth or Barry Bonds? Johnny Unitas or Peyton Manning? Jessie Owens or Carl Lewis? Michael Jordan or Kobe Bryant? Or was it Elgin Baylor? Butkus or Singletary? The debates could go on forever.

Boyer Coe says Sergio Oliva had the most impressive performance ever in 1971—and he didn't even win. But I'd have to say the top three are Arnold, Lee, and Ronnie. I would then pick Lee as the greatest because I think his eight straight wins were accomplished against the most intense competition. Shawn Ray agrees with me. Lou Ferrigno, who might have won a couple titles if he hadn't gone into acting, says you could flip a coin between Arnold and Ronnie. So I know not everyone agrees with me, and there are so many variables and hypotheticals that any discussion of "who's the greatest?" is just for fun.

What's important for me to remember, even at age 48, is to be the best I can be. It's a great reminder for you too—be the best you can be in relation to your goals. That's all that counts!

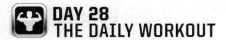

DAY 28
THE DAILY WORKOUT

THE MUSCLE BUILDER: REST

HARDGAINER WORKOUT: REST

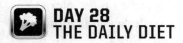

DAY 28
THE DAILY DIET

MEAL 1: Myofusion Shake: 2 scoops Myofusion, 1/2 cup egg whites, 2/3 cup instant oatmeal, 1 tablespoon natural peanut butter or almond butter, 1/2 cup apple juice, 1/2 cup water and ice.

MEAL 2: Myofusion Protein Pancakes: 1 scoop Myofusion, 1 cup egg whites, 1 cup oatmeal, 1/4 cup chopped walnuts, 1 sliced banana. Mix all together and cook on low heat on a non-stick pan using cooking spray. Optional: add sugar-free syrup.

MEAL 3: Same as Meal 1.

MEAL 4: 8 ounces of lean steak, 1 sweet potato, 1 cup asparagus.

MEAL 5: Same as Meal 1.

MEAL 6: 8 ounces grilled chicken breast, 1 cup brown rice, 1 cup steamed broccoli.

MEAL 7 *[optional]*: Same as Meal 1.

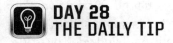

DAY 28
THE DAILY TIP

To try and fail is but to learn; to fail to try is to suffer the painful regret of what might have been.

DAY 29 HOW TO RIDE THE ROLLER COASTER

If there's one thing I've learned, it's that life is not a straight line. It's not a Kansas highway where you can put the car in cruise control, take a nap, and wake up in Colorado. If you're driving a car there will be potholes and some crazy drivers, including the person who cuts you off in heavy traffic while eating a sandwich, looking for a better radio station, and texting their BFF.

Now we can cause some of our own adversity through bad choices and behaviors. If you don't show up to work on time for the entire week, there's no one else to blame but yourself for getting fired. Some adversity comes our way through the bad choices of others. If your dad was an alcoholic, there's a good chance you had a tough childhood because of his problems. Some adversity just seems to be a matter of bad luck. Insurance agents have a term in most policies, *force majeure*, that describes what appears to be acts of God—floods, hurricanes, earthquakes, and other huge calamities that just happen.

You can eliminate some adversity by making consistent and good choices. But there will still be lows in life. If the roller coaster goes up, it is bound to go down. You already know firsthand that life holds some adversity. We all know it. But surprisingly, we still get blindsided by it. We all know people who freak out when things don't go their way, big or small.

If you work out hard, I guarantee you will get hurt from time to time. On a rainy day, my left shoulder reminds me how hard I trained when I was young and thought I was indestructible. If you are in a relationship or have a significant other, I guarantee there won't be candlelight and roses on the table every night. There will be some fights and disagreements. Doesn't mean you don't love each other. It means you're human. If you are a parent, I guarantee your kids aren't going to respond to everything you want them to do in the way you think they should—even when you think you are being perfectly reasonable and fair. If you own your own business, I guarantee there will be months and quarters and situations when you wish the buck didn't stop with you.

So how do you ride the roller coaster of life? I think there's an underused and underrated word that is such a huge determinant of your overall success: *poise*. When you're poised, it's almost like you knew trouble was coming before it got there and when everyone else was whining and complaining you were handling what needed to be handled. Poise is a little bit like a duck crossing a pond. On the surface, it seems to glide effortlessly across the water, but what no one can see is that beneath the surface, those webbed feet are churning like crazy.

Poise is an attitude of optimism. It knows that no problem is big enough to conquer you. It brings wisdom and patience to the table. Someone mouths off at you and instead of lashing out and escalating things, you ignore what needs to be ignored. You are poised when you get a grip on your temper. Poise isn't meek and it doesn't mean you don't have passion and emotions—believe me, or I would have no poise at all. But it's a tool of self-control that marshals your strengths to handle whatever life throws at you.

I won bodybuilding contests due to poise. I overcame adversity due to poise. I lead a successful company due to poise. It's the only way I know how to ride the roller coaster called life. Next time some adversity comes your way make it an opportunity—raise your game.

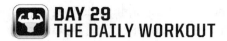

DAY 29
THE DAILY WORKOUT

THE MUSCLE BUILDER: CHEST & ABS
(Take 45 seconds - 1 minute rest between each set)
Incline dumbbell press – 4 sets of 8-10 reps
Incline dumbbell flies – 4 sets of 8-10 reps
Decline cable flies – 4 sets of 8-10 reps
Superset: Dumbbell flat bench, Pec Dec – 4 sets of 8-10 reps
Crunches – 4 sets of 25-30 reps
Leg raises – 4 sets of 25-30 reps

CARDIO
20-30 minutes interval cardio on treadmill

HARDGAINER WORKOUT: CHEST/BACK/BICEPS/TRICEPS/CORE
Modified Compound Superset #1 – *Take 45 seconds rest before
moving on to the 2nd exercise*
Incline Dumbbell Press: 3 sets of 6-8 reps (45 Sec Rest)
Barbell Bent Over Row: 3 sets of 6-8 reps (1 min rest)
Modified Compound Superset #2 – *Take 45 seconds rest before
moving on to the 2nd exercise*
Flat Dumbbell Bench Press: 3 sets of 6-8 reps (45 Sec Rest)
Chin-Ups: 3 sets of 6-8 reps (Strap on weight if you can)(1 min rest)
*Note: If you cannot perform the Chin-up, either have someone spot
you by using your legs off their hands for leverage or have them
spot-push you up by the waist.*
Superset #3 – *No rest between exercises*
Barbell Curls: 3 sets of 8-10 reps (No Rest)
Close Grip Dumbbell Bench Press (Triceps): 3 sets of 8-10 reps
(1 min rest)
Superset #4 – *No rest between exercises*
Dumbbell Hammer Curls: 3 sets of 10-12 reps (No Rest)
Triceps Pushdowns: 3 sets of 10-12 reps (1 min rest)
Superset #4 – *No rest between exercises*
Plank: 2 sets of 1 Minute Static Contraction (No Rest)
Bicycle Maneuver: 2 sets of 30 reps (1 min rest)

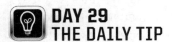 **DAY 29**
THE DAILY DIET

MEAL 1: Myofusion Shake: 2 scoops Myofusion, 1/2 cup egg whites, 2/3 cup instant oatmeal, 1 tablespoon natural peanut butter or almond butter, 1/2 cup apple juice, 1/2 cup water and ice.

MEAL 2: Myofusion Protein Pancakes: 1 scoop Myofusion, 1 cup egg whites, 1 cup oatmeal, 1/4 cup chopped walnuts, 1 sliced banana. Mix all together and cook on low heat on a non-stick pan using cooking spray. Optional: add sugar-free syrup.

MEAL 3: Same as Meal 1.

MEAL 4: Egg omelet: 1 cup egg whites mixed with 1 cup chopped peppers, onions, and tomatoes. 1 slice watermelon on the side.

MEAL 5: 10 raw almonds.

MEAL 6: 8 ounces mahi mahi or other white fish, 1 small potato, 3 ounces steamed string beans, 4 ounce green salad with vinegar.

MEAL 7 [optional]**:** Same as Meal 1.

DAY 29
THE DAILY TIP

When you do bench presses, switch the angle of the bench and the width of your grips. This makes sure you are giving every area of your chest attention.

DAY 30 APPEARANCES MATTER—SOMETIMES

If I told you appearances don't matter, you'd call me a liar. You know by now that by virtue of me being a bodybuilder that I love appearances. From age 13 on, I've dedicated myself to maximizing my appearance. The biggest muscles possible. The most vascularity. Symmetry. Ripped definition. I've gone so far as to let others judge my appearance. I jest, because you know that judges ultimately declare winners and runner-ups at bodybuilding contests. But I've let the general population judge my appearance, too, with all my magazine appearances. One thing you learn early on as a bodybuilder is that not everyone says nice things about you. I have no problem with the fact that some people just don't like big muscles. I suspect a few negative assessments likely come from people with just a little bit of jealousy.

Appearance matters in business, too. Because I have a supplement company focused on helping people attain their ultimate body, I don't have the same requirements or standards of performance as a banker or lawyer—though every now and then I do have to dress up. When people I work with see me dressed up in a navy blue business suit with a power tie they kid me and ask if I'm going to see the banker or going to a funeral. Back in the early days of launching a company either place would have felt about the same! But my point is, I know appearance matters and so do you. You bought this book and are in the program to improve how you look. You might be trying to impress a particular member of the opposite sex or you might just want to look great for all the world to see. That's great.

But sometimes appearances don't matter. The most pointed criticisms of me throughout my career as a pro bodybuilder and then businessman have focused on some of my personality traits: I hustle; I'm always enthusiastic; I don't mind getting my hands dirty to get the job done. Now I'm going to keep it clean and not tell anyone that they can kiss my glutes, but I have to tell you, if the worst thing anyone says about you is that you are over-the-top enthusiastic, tell whoever said it thanks for the compliment and don't change a thing.

Some people are too cool to compete and lose. I took 6th in my first youth event and 5th in my first national event. You have to start somewhere and I'm proud of both of those finishes. Some people are too cool to take a job they feel is beneath their dignity. I'm of the opinion that honest work is honorable. I think people worry too much about being "underemployed." It may be true. But hard work gets things fixed over time. I'm glad I'm not selling my supplements out of the back of my trunk anymore. But I couldn't have gotten to where I am any other way.

Hey, if you're laid back and cool—that's cool with me. I simply want to stress that it's okay to be yourself. Not just okay—it's the only way to be. The judgments and criticisms of others can be helpful in life. You just have to know when those opinions matter—and when they don't. If criticism has truth to it and can help you perform better in any area of life, by all means receive it with gratitude—even if it pisses you off a little. But when criticism is more about the other person's negativity than anything you've done or not done just let it slide off your back. Don't let them get under your skin or rob you of who you are.

That takes self-confidence and wisdom. We won't get it right every time. But knowing there's a time to listen and a time to ignore is the first part in getting it right.

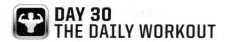

DAY 30
THE DAILY WORKOUT

THE MUSCLE BUILDER: BACK & CALVES
(Take 45 seconds - 1 minute rest between each set)

Deadlifts – 4 sets of 8-10 reps
Wide grip chins – 4 sets of 8-10 reps
Superset: Close grip pulldowns, Wide grip cable pullovers – 4 sets of 8-10 reps
Superset: Cable low rows, T-bar rows – 4 sets of 8-10 reps
Superset: Two arm dumbbell rows, machine rows – 4 sets of 8-10 reps
Standing Calf raises – 5 sets of 15 reps
Seated calf raises – 5 sets of 15 reps

CARDIO

20-30 minutes interval cardio on treadmill

HARDGAINER WORKOUT:THIGHS/HAMSTRINGS/DELTS/CALVES/LOWER ABS

Superset #1
Wide Stance Squats: 3 sets of 4-6 reps (45 Seconds Rest)
Stiff Legged Barbell Deadlifts: 3 sets of 4-6 reps (1 min rest)

> *Note: Utilize the "Full Body Tension Technique": This is when you stay in proper anatomical form and maintain that posture by keeping all of your major muscles contracted before and throughout the movements. This will keep you safe, while allowing you to use maximum intensity.*

Giant Set #2 – *3 exercises performed back-to-back without rest*
Leg Press: 3 sets of 6-8 reps (No Rest)
Leg Extensions: 3 sets of 10-12 reps (No Rest)
Lying Leg Curls: 3 sets of 10-12 reps (1 min rest)
Giant Set #3
Upright Barbell Row: 3 sets of 8-10 reps (No Rest)
Lateral Raises: 3 sets of 8-10 reps (No Rest)
Descending Set #4 – *Drop the weight as you move from set–to-set*
Standing Calf Raises (Gastrocs) - 3 Descending Sets – Decrease weight

as you descend, if necessary:
- 1st set of 12-15 reps (15 sec rest)
- 2nd set of 12-15 reps (15 sec rest)
- 3rd set of 12-15 reps (1 min rest & repeat 2 more times)

Superset #5
Bent Over Lateral Dumbbell Raises: 3 sets of 10-12 reps (No Rest)
Seated Calf Raises (Soleus): 3 sets of 10-12 reps (1 min rest)
Hanging Leg Raises: 3 sets of 15-20 reps (1 min rest)

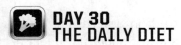

DAY 30
THE DAILY DIET

MEAL 1: Myofusion Shake: 2 scoops Myofusion, 1/2 cup egg whites, 2/3 cup instant oatmeal, 1 tablespoon natural peanut butter or almond butter, 1/2 cup apple juice, 1/2 cup water and ice.

MEAL 2: Myofusion Protein Pancakes: 1 scoop Myofusion, 1 cup egg whites, 1 cup oatmeal, 1/4 cup chopped walnuts, 1 sliced banana. Mix all together and cook on low heat on a non-stick pan using cooking spray. Optional: add sugar-free syrup.

MEAL 3: 10 raw almonds.

MEAL 4: 8 ounces grilled chicken breast, 1 cup brown rice, 1 banana.

MEAL 5: Same as Meal 1.

MEAL 6: 8 ounces lean ground beef, 1 cup gluten-free pasta, 4-6 ounces low sodium natural tomato sauce with 1 tablespoon grated cheese (optional), 4 ounces green salad with vinegar.

MEAL 7 (optional): Same as Meal 1.

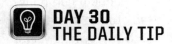

DAY 30
THE DAILY TIP

Whether you're performing a seated cable row, a one-arm dumbbell row, or a pull-up, try to squeeze your shoulder blades together as you lift the weight on every rep. Heavy weight, concentration, and a super intense mid-point contraction during your reps will bring on far better results than simply trying to move max weight from point A to point B.

DAY 31 TEST EVERYTHING

Even with laws that require truth in advertising, we all know that not everything we are told about a product or program is true. It was P.T. Barnum that said, "There's a sucker born every minute." None of us like to be played for a fool. But some of us still don't take the time to check out what we're being sold. From insurance to investments to healthcare products to political promises, it appears P.T. Barnum was right. There's a lot of suckers out there.

I know what I am about to say sounds like a commercial. If that warning makes you suspicious of what you are about to read, good. I'm already making my point. So even with that warning, what I'm about to say is something I believe with all my heart—and there's an important life lesson I want you to pick up. After I retired from competition over a decade ago as an IFBB Hall of Fame athlete, I knew I loved the sport far too much to walk away. I had to stay involved, but wasn't sure which avenue I would take. Then it came to me. What if I took the same work ethic and never-say-die attitude that had taken me so far battling it out on stage and focused it on a supplement company?

I certainly felt I knew what it took to make dramatic changes to the human form through my own physique as well as those I had mentored. Again, people told me to forget about it. I was a small-timer out of New Jersey up against established multimillion-dollar companies and I couldn't compete with that. They should have known better than to tell me that—it only makes me want to achieve that "impossible" goal even more.

Now, 16 years later, Gaspari Nutrition has grown into one of the leaders in the supplement industry. Why? The obvious reason is that our products really work. I simply thought that if I was to make products better than anyone had ever done before and sponsor the unbiased, independent research to prove it, I couldn't go wrong. And I already knew that the most important sell was the second sell. When you buy a product and it does exactly what you hoped it would, you tend to buy it again. You're also likely to recommend the product to others. And, you're probably going to try any new products that company makes.

With all of the effort you put into building your physique, trying to figure out which supplements are worth the investment shouldn't be an added strain on your time. Every athlete should be availed the opportunity to maximize his or her efforts with the best supplements available. Learn as much as you can, check the sources of your information, and the truth will reveal itself.

There are two words I want you to highlight in your mind: independent research. I have personally participated in the development and testing of every product we create. I even went so far as to earn certification from the National Institute of Sports Medicine. But you know what? That wasn't good enough for me. So what I started doing early in my company's history was funding area universities to conduct independent, scientific research on my products so I could back up my claims from science. There's a history of "snake oil" in my industry and I wanted to rise above that.

My commitment and passion goes way back to my first days as a bodybuilder. I don't know of any other bodybuilder who kept more detailed notes on every aspect of their training, from workouts to meals to sleep and to supplements. I kept track of my progress in meeting my goals and studied my journal to see what was happening to help or hurt. I couldn't isolate independent variables every time, but I got pretty good at knowing what worked and what didn't work for me. In essence, I was running independent research on the methods and supplements available to me at each period of time I was training.

Over the course of these 51 days, I've given you a lot to think about. I hope you've paid attention to what I have to say. But check out for yourself what I'm telling you to do. If what works for me needs to be fine-tuned for your physiology, don't give a second thought to making adjustments. Once again, I want to encourage you to keep up with your journal. Take it with you everywhere. If you're behind on charting your workouts, food, supplements, rest, and progress, then now is the time to get caught up.

You may not be interested in becoming an expert on sports medicine and nutrition. But you do need to become an expert on what works best for you. There's only one way to do that. Test everything!

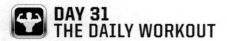

DAY 31
THE DAILY WORKOUT

THE MUSCLE BUILDER: LEGS
(Take 45 seconds - 1 minute rest between each set)
Lying leg curls – 5 sets of 10-12 reps
Stiff-legged deadlifts – 4 sets of 10-12 reps
Leg extensions – 5 sets of 10-12 reps (double drop set on last set)
45-degree Leg Press – 4 sets of 15 reps (double drop set on last set)
Hack Squat – 3 sets of 15 reps (triple drop set on last set)
Superset: Squats, walking lunges – 3 sets of 15-20 reps

CARDIO
20-30 minutes interval cardio on treadmill

HARDGAINER WORKOUT: REST

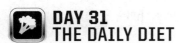

DAY 31
THE DAILY DIET

MEAL 1: Myofusion Shake: 2 scoops Myofusion, 1/2 cup egg whites, 2/3 cup instant oatmeal, 1 tablespoon natural peanut butter or almond butter, 1/2 cup apple juice, 1/2 cup water and ice.
MEAL 2: Myofusion Protein Pancakes: 1 scoop Myofusion, 1 cup egg whites, 1 cup oatmeal, 1/4 cup chopped walnuts, 1 sliced banana. Mix all together and cook on low heat on a non-stick pan using cooking spray. Optional: add sugar-free syrup.
MEAL 3: Same as Meal 1.
MEAL 4: 1 cup tuna salad, 1 cup brown rice, 6 ounces green salad with vinegar.
MEAL 5: 4 brown rice cakes.
MEAL 6: 6 ounces lean buffalo patty *(or 93% lean ground beef)* with salsa or mustard, 1 sweet potato, 1 cup asparagus.
MEAL 7 *(optional)*: Same as Meal 1.

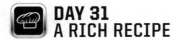

DAY 31
A RICH RECIPE

TUNA SALAD

12 ounces grilled tuna

1 large, sweet red apple, chopped

2 tablespoons lemon juice

1/4 cup orange juice

2 large bell peppers, chopped

2 large stalks celery, chopped

2 small red onions, chopped

2 tablespoons olive oil

3 tablespoons red wine vinegar

sea salt and ground black pepper to taste

Gently toss all ingredients in a large bowl. Serve chilled.

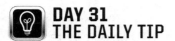

DAY 31
THE DAILY TIP

As people become more conscious of health and fitness, new products reach the market. Had you heard of Greek yogurt even three or four years ago? It has better fat and probiotics than regular yogurt. I love mixing it with a little granola and a fruit like blueberries or bananas for a great snack.

DAY 32 IS YOUR NETWORK UP AND RUNNING?

My story tends to focus a lot on what I have accomplished individually and on my own personality traits. My determination. My work ethic. My resilience. My physique. My victories. My company.

Along the way I hope you have heard me speak loud and clear about the many people who have contributed so much to everything I've been able to do. Legends like Joe Gold, Ed Connors, and Arnold Schwarzenegger. Friends and rivals like Lee Haney, Ronnie Coleman, Samir Bannout, and Chris Cormier. I've talked about the power of teamwork within my company, and the wisdom of hiring people that do certain things better and smarter than me.

Nothing makes me as thankful as my family. How great to grow up with parents who were very firm but very loving. To have a brother who took me in when I was flat broke.

If you are struggling to make headway in your drive to achieve your ultimate body—and your ultimate you—take a few minutes to evaluate your network. Is it time for a personal trainer? I've mentioned that I never had a coach. I learned from books and trial and error. But I want to underscore right now that in that specific regard, my experience is probably the exception and not the rule. We love the exceptions in business and sports, but we are wiser to manage and bet with rules.

Do you have someone older and wiser to mentor you

in your career? Do you have someone younger in your life who you are helping to grow? We all need someone to help and someone to help us. Do you have friends who build you up or tear you down? How about your relationship with your parents? No doubt they aren't perfect and maybe you had a rough upbringing. But we only grow when we stretch ourselves to reach out to those who are most important in our lives. I loved my dad like crazy—and he drove me crazy. I still wanted to make him proud.

I know this is heavy stuff. But writing this book has invigorated me. It's made me do some serious reflection in order to put these words on a page. I've said from the introduction and throughout the book, this is about more than an ultimate body. It's about the ultimate you. As I talk about me and challenge you with what you need to do, don't forget to check your network and upgrade where necessary.

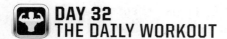

DAY 32
THE DAILY WORKOUT

THE MUSCLE BUILDER: SHOULDERS & ABS
(Take 45 seconds - 1 minute rest between each set)

Seated barbell front press – 4 sets of 8-12 reps

Giantset: Seated side laterals, Arnold Press, Standing dumbbell upright rows – 4 sets of 10-12 reps

Incline one arm side laterals – 3 sets of 12-15

Machine rear laterals – 4 sets of 12-15

Barbell shrugs from behind – 4 sets of 12-15

Twisting crunches – 4 sets of 30 reps

Leg raises – 4 sets of 25 reps

CARDIO
20-30 minutes interval cardio on treadmill

HARDGAINER WORKOUT: CHEST/BACK/BICEPS/TRICEPS/ABS

Modified Compound Superset #1

Flat Dumbbell Bench Press: 3 sets of 8, 6, 4 reps (90 second rest)

Close Grip Neutral Grip Pull-Ups: 3 sets of 8, 6, 4 reps (Strap weight on if you can – 2 mins rest)

> *Note: If you cannot perform the Close Grip Pull-Up, either have someone spot you by using your legs off their hands for leverage or have them spot-push you up by the waist.*

Modified Compound Superset #2

Incline Barbell Bench Press: 3 sets of 8, 6, 4 reps (90 second rest)

Bent Over Underhand Barbell Row: 3 sets of 8, 6, 4 reps (2 min rest)

Giant Modified Compound Super Set #3 – *Take prescribed rest between exercise*

Chest Dips: 3 sets of 8, 6, 4 reps (60 second rest)

Preacher Curls: 3 sets of 8, 6, 4 reps (45 second rest)

Close Grip Bench Press: 3 sets of 8, 6, 4 reps (2 min rest)

Giant Modified Compound Super Set #4

E-Z Preacher Curls: 3 sets of 8, 6, 4 reps (60 second rest)

Lying Triceps Extensions: 3 sets of 8, 6, 4 reps (45 second rest)
Swiss Ball (aka "Inflated Fitness Ball") Crunches: 3 sets of 20, 15,
 10 reps (Hold a weight plate or dumbbell overhead if you can)
 (2 min rest)

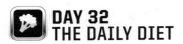

DAY 32
THE DAILY DIET

MEAL 1: Myofusion Shake: 2 scoops Myofusion, 1/2 cup egg whites, 2/3
 cup instant oatmeal, 1 tablespoon natural peanut butter or
 almond butter, 1/2 cup apple juice, 1/2 cup water and ice.
MEAL 2: Myofusion Protein Pancakes: 1 scoop Myofusion, 1 cup egg
 whites, 1 cup oatmeal, 1/4 cup chopped walnuts, 1 sliced
 banana. Mix all together and cook on low heat on a non-stick
 pan using cooking spray. Optional: add sugar-free syrup.
MEAL 3: Same as Meal 1.
MEAL 4: 6 ounces grilled chicken breast, 1 cup brown rice, 1 apple.
MEAL 5: 10 raw almonds.
MEAL 6: 8 ounces grilled chicken breast, 1 cup quinoa, 3 ounces
 steamed string beans, 4 ounces green salad with vinegar.
MEAL 7 *(optional)*: 2 scoops of Myofusion, 1/2 cup apple juice,
 1 tablespoon natural peanut butter.

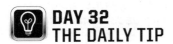

DAY 32
THE DAILY TIP

*You don't have to do endless repetitions to get great abs. Slow down. Do
full-range movements. Progressive-resistance workouts are great for
development and the best results.*

DAY 33 FAT BOY

One of the nicknames I was given at the beginning of my career was Fat Boy. That's what Lee Haney called me when we first met. I had just moved to California. Ed Connors recruited me to manage one of his Gold's Gyms. The pay wasn't great but he sweetened the deal by giving a few points so I had an equity stake in the gym. I wasn't the only one he did this for. He liked to hire young guys who came to California to take their bodybuilding career to the next level because he knew it would attract serious customers. He wanted his gyms to be the place where serious lifting and training was taking place. I really didn't have to attract anyone to the Gold's Gym I managed. It was already full of major players. For example, the other manager was a man named Steve Borden. He would later go on to achieve great fame as the professional wrestler known as Sting.

That's where I met Albert Beckles. He had a longer journey to arrive in California than I did. He was born in Barbados but started his bodybuilding career in England. He came to the U.S. to turn pro and in 1971 he won the IFBB Mr. Universe title. He set the record for most appearances in the Mr. Olympia contest. It's hard to believe he was able to compete in that thirteen times—he placed in the top five six different times. He came in second to Lee Haney twice. That's the kind of worker he was.

Cory Everson worked out there, too. She was one of the first female bodybuilding superstars and won Ms.

Olympia six years in a row. She got her start back in Madison, Wisconsin, where she was a multi-sport star for the Badgers. Jeff Everson, a great competitive bodybuilder, was her trainer and when the two got married and came to California, her career took off. I could go on and on with a who's who list that trained there.

Another Mr. Universe, Bertil Fox, also originally from the West Indies, trained there. Tom Platz, Fred Hatfields, Hulk Hogan, Steve Borden, Lee Haney, Cory Everson, Jeff Everson, Bertal Fox, Tom Platz, Fred Hatfields, James Brian Hellwig, better known to the wrestling world as the Ultimate Warrior. He was an intense worker and was a great physical specimen. Rick Wayne was there. Born on the island of St. Lucia, he was a pop singer and a professional bodybuilder, but is famous now as a great writer, editor, and TV personality where he is always fighting government corruption. I hate to name names because I'm leaving so many out. I'm not even starting on the Hollywood actors who showed up there.

Enter a 255-pound kid from New Jersey named Rich Gaspari. I was one strong dude. As part of my workouts I would squat 775 pounds, bench 520 pounds, and do curls with 200 pound barbells. I was strong as anyone in there, but not necessarily impressive with my physique. I think I had 30 or 40 pounds of fat. I was still eating a dozen eggs, drinking a gallon of milk, and downing a jar of peanut butter every day. I thought I had to bulk up as much as possible if I was going to have enough mass to compete against naturally larger competitors. So every time I competed, I had to starve myself to show any cuts. That's why Lee gave me the nickname Fat Boy.

He basically changed everything about my training. He got me to improve my diet dramatically. I cut out a lot of the fat. I started eating more often—and yes, at least a little protein every meal. I had already suffered a number of injuries due to the amount of weights I was lifting. Lee got me to cut back and taught me that the muscle doesn't know weight—only failure. You don't have to bench more than 500 pounds to take your chest muscles to failure. My form was bad and I was jerking the weights to move them. He got me to slow down and squeeze the muscle on every rep. The results were immediate and dramatic.

He taught me to stimulate—not annihilate—my muscles.

I was always a hard worker, but my training strategy wasn't focused on anything but using brute strength. Lee taught me to channel my limitless energy—he claimed I was foaming at the mouth when it was workout time—and my enthusiasm into great form. Not only did I achieve greater success earlier than anyone thought was possible, I got rid of the nickname Fat Boy and became known as the Dragon Slayer.

Slow down. Yes—work hard today. But focus on form. Squeeze every rep and get everything you can out of your workout. Your muscles will thank you!

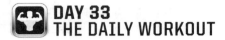 **DAY 33**
THE DAILY WORKOUT

THE MUSCLE BUILDER: BICEPS & TRICEPS
(Take 45 seconds - 1 minute rest between each set)

Superset: Incline dumbbell curls, Rope pushdowns – 4 sets of 10 reps
Superset: Standing barbell curls, Seated 2-arm overhead tricep extension with Dumbbell – 4 sets of 10 reps
Superset: Seated preacher curls with EZ curl bar, Lying pullover press – 4 sets of 10 reps
Superset: Dumbbell concentration curls, cable kickbacks – 4 sets of 10 reps

CARDIO
20-30 minutes interval cardio on treadmill

HARDGAINER WORKOUT: THIGHS/HAMSTRINGS/DELTS/CALVES
Modified Compound Superset #1
Medium Stance Squats: 3 sets of 8, 6, 4 reps (90 second rest)
Lying Leg Curls: 3 sets of 8, 6, 4 reps (90 second rest)

> *Note: If you suffer from lower back problems you may substitute the squat for the leg press. Since you are performing the leg press as your second exercise, then just use a close stance on this one and a medium stance on the second one.*

Modified Compound Superset #2
Leg Press: 3 sets of 8, 6, 4 reps (90 second rest)
Barbell Romanian Deadlifts: 3 sets of 8, 6, 4 reps (2 min rest)
Modified Compound Superset #3
Seated Barbell Front Shoulder: 3 sets of 8, 6, 4 reps (60 second rest)
Standing Calf Raise (Gastrocs): 3 sets of 10, 8, 6 reps (2 min rest)
Modified Compound Superset #4
Dumbbell Lateral Raises: 3 sets of 8, 6, 4 reps (60 second rest)
Lying Leg Raises with a pop at the top of each rep: 3 sets of 10, 8, 6 reps (60 second rest)
Descending Set #5 – *Drop the weight as you move from set-to-set*

Seated Calf Raises (Soleus) - 3 Descending Sets – Decrease weight as you descend, if necessary:
  • 1st set of 12-15 reps (15 sec rest)
  • 2nd set of 12-15 reps (15 sec rest)
  • 3rd set of 12-15 reps (1 min rest & repeat 2 more times)

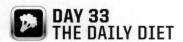

DAY 33
THE DAILY DIET

MEAL 1: Myofusion Shake: 2 scoops Myofusion, 1/2 cup egg whites, 2/3 cup instant oatmeal, 1 tablespoon natural peanut butter or almond butter, 1/2 cup apple juice, 1/2 cup water and ice.

MEAL 2: Myofusion Protein Pancakes: 1 scoop Myofusion, 1 cup egg whites, 1 cup oatmeal, 1/4 cup chopped walnuts, 1 sliced banana. Mix all together and cook on low heat on a non-stick pan using cooking spray. Optional: add sugar-free syrup.

MEAL 3: Same as Meal 1.

MEAL 4: 8 ounces grilled chicken breast, 1 cup brown rice, 1 cup steamed broccoli.

MEAL 5: 10 raw almonds.

MEAL 6: 1 cup egg whites mixed with 1 cup chopped peppers, onions, and tomatoes, 1 slice watermelon.

MEAL 7 *(optional)*: Same as Meal 1.

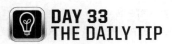

DAY 33
THE DAILY TIP

My arms were a stubborn gainer for me and were holding me back. I went with less weight and better form and got my arms up to 20.5 inches. Not bad. If you have stubborn areas, it takes some experimentation to find what works!

DAY 34 ARE YOU TEACHABLE?

After about four months in California, I quit the job managing a Gold's Gym to become a trainer. With the Hollywood crowd out there, I could make more money and the hours were more flexible so I could focus on my own training. One of my favorite clients was Robert Blake, a popular actor who had played a quirky detective in the television show *Baretta*. He was from the East Coast so he liked having a Jersey kid as his trainer. He talked me up a lot to his friends and probably sent me more new business than anyone else.

When I bought my gym in New Jersey after retiring as a pro, I was a trainer again. If the gym had been financially successful maybe I would still be a trainer today. Although even then I realized there was a huge need for education on supplements. I don't believe we can get all the nutrition it takes to build a huge body on food alone. Oliva did it as a vegetarian—but he has to be the rarest of exceptions. So in some form or another I would have been in the supplement business, but I'm sure on a vastly smaller scale.

I've been asked if I liked being a trainer. The answer is absolutely yes. And the answer is absolutely no. I was and am too intense and passionate about training to be content as a "trophy trainer." It was more the case in California, but even in New Jersey, when the fitness craze was booming, there were a lot of clients who wanted their own trainer to brag to their friends about. I'm just not wired to smile and be Mr. Encouragement when it is workout time. I walk into a gym and a switch goes off in my brain. I don't cuss and swear at people, but I still take on the persona of a drill sergeant. I'm not doing it for show. It really does come from my heart.

So I love working with people at all levels of physical achievement as long as they are teachable. Being teachable doesn't just mean listening, watching, and understanding what is being taught. It means doing it. Head knowledge is great, but the one who is applying that knowledge is the one who is really learning. If someone had a body area that was underdeveloped and that caused them problems on form and performance, I had all the patience in the world helping them to walk before they ran—as long as they tried. Well, as long as they tried hard.

But I have to be honest. I couldn't stand training people who just weren't into it, who were going through the motions. Six months into working with me they still couldn't do a curl right. They hadn't changed their diet. I could tell they didn't sleep much. They wanted to chat about their week, not just before and after the session but in the middle of training. If you aren't sweating and breathing heavy enough to make talking difficult if not impossible, it's time to push a little harder. If I had made a career as a full trainer I might have blown a gasket over time. That's why I sometimes suspect that the best thing that ever happened to me was failing miserably as a gym owner.

I don't care how many bodybuilding books you buy or how many hours you spend in the gym each week. Knowledge and hours don't mean anything if you aren't teachable—if you aren't really working the plan. There's a few reading this who have followed the workouts I've outlined but still have never taken a muscle to the point of absolute fatigue. Some look at the list and think, *This is pretty easy*. That's only because they are making it easy. They really haven't learned what I'm proposing here. They aren't teachable yet.

There's an old Chinese proverb that says, "When the student is ready, the teacher will arrive." In other words, even if Aristotle is your logic professor and Arnold is your trainer—until you are really ready to learn you won't recognize a great teacher right in front of you.

Are you teachable? You ready to do things different than before? Are you ready to walk the walk?

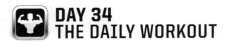 **DAY 34**
THE DAILY WORKOUT

THE MUSCLE BUILDER: REST

HARDGAINER WORKOUT: REST

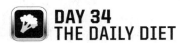 **DAY 34**
THE DAILY DIET

MEAL 1: Myofusion Shake: 2 scoops Myofusion, 1/2 cup egg whites, 2/3 cup instant oatmeal, 1 tablespoon natural peanut butter or almond butter, 1/2 cup apple juice, 1/2 cup water and ice.

MEAL 2: Myofusion Protein Pancakes: 1 scoop Myofusion, 1 cup egg whites, 1 cup oatmeal, 1/4 cup chopped walnuts, 1 sliced banana. Mix all together and cook on low heat on a non-stick pan using cooking spray. Optional: add sugar-free syrup.

MEAL 3: Same as Meal 1.

MEAL 4: 8 ounces grilled chicken mixed with 1 cup brown rice, 1 tablespoon olive oil or salad dressing with 1 cup fresh veggies.

MEAL 5: Same as Meal 1.

MEAL 6: 8 ounces lean ground beef, 1 cup gluten-free pasta, 4-6 ounces low sodium natural tomato sauce with 1 tablespoon grated cheese [optional].

MEAL 7 [optional]**:** Same as Meal 1.

DAY 34
THE DAILY TIP

What's the best way to fuel your workout? When it comes to weight training, you need carbohydrates—they deliver the optimum focus and high-octane energy you need. Starving yourself or training on empty will only exhaust you and lead to a crappy workout. Stick with foods like bananas, whole grain bread, low-fat yogurt with berries mixed in, steel cut oatmeal, and sweet potatoes. These are great sources of carbs which will convert to muscle glycogen to keep those muscles ready to work.

DAY 35 DON'T SETTLE!

Time to do some honest self-assessment. Are you training your body like never before or are you settling for what you've always done? One definition of insanity is doing the same things over and over and expecting different results. Are you wanting your ultimate body without doing your ultimate program? I'm sorry, it's not going to happen. No offense, but you're crazy if you think it works that way.

We live in a culture that can be very self-indulgent. There are a lot of lazy people. We like things easy. Is it any wonder there is so much mediocrity? We have rampant obesity among youth and adults alike. People want to blame fast food companies. But they are only giving us what we demand. No one is going to get after you if you hit the gym and just go about what you were doing before. Heck, some people will say what you are doing is incredible. But someone close to you knows better than to feel good about a so-so effort. It's not your spouse or parent or best friend that isn't going to be proud of you. That someone is you.

I love the quote by Johann Wolfgang von Goethe: "Dream no small dreams for they have no power to move the hearts of men." The only thing I would say to you is forget moving the hearts of others. Why not stir your own heart? Deciding to go to the gym and doing a half-assed circuit on the exercise machines might be good enough for someone else. But what about you?

If you settle for middle of the road effort and results, don't forget you are as close to the bottom as you are to the top. Is that what you want? Do you want the epithet on your gravestone to read, "Better than half the population!"

The surest way to kill your dreams is by giving a half-hearted effort. Giving less than your best only makes you feel bad about yourself, so instead of striving and reaching higher, you lower the standards. If you shoot an arrow and then draw a circle around wherever it lands, I guess you can tell people you hit the bulls eye every time. But someone knows you aren't being true to yourself. And that someone is you.

How do you rekindle a flame that has basically blown out? You can watch a movie like *300* or *Gladiator* or *Braveheart* or *Remember the Titans*. You can get on my website and watch some great videos on effort and technique. If you have never watched my *Walk the Walk* series, do so. It will help fire you up. You can load your iPod with some great songs. All those things might help. But ultimately you are going to have to hit the gym and do exactly what you set out to do. You are going to have to go an entire day eating exactly what is prescribed. You are going to have to tell your friends you aren't going clubbing because you have to catch a full eight hours of sleep. Success breeds success. Nothing feels better than doing exactly what you determined to do—no matter how hard and painful it might be. In fact the harder it was the better you feel. The old adage is still true: No pain, no gain.

But, Rich . . . .

Nope. Stop right there. I'm not even listening this time. No excuses. I don't want to hear them. And guess what? Neither do you. I'm doing you a favor by telling you to shut up and save it.

It's time to walk the walk. It's time to slay a dragon. It's time to get fierce. How do you start? You do it today. That's all you have to worry about. Today. Do everything better and harder than you ever have before. Do that and tomorrow will take care of itself.

I'd close this with something inspiring and motivational but I don't want to. I don't want to give you anything. I want you to go out and take whatever it is you are supposed to have today with your own determination and self-motivation.

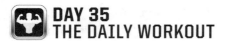 **DAY 35**
THE DAILY WORKOUT

THE MUSCLE BUILDER: REST

HARDGAINER WORKOUT: REST

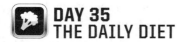 **DAY 35**
THE DAILY DIET

MEAL 1: Myofusion Shake: 2 scoops Myofusion, 1/2 cup egg whites, 2/3 cup instant oatmeal, 1 tablespoon natural peanut butter or almond butter, 1/2 cup apple juice, 1/2 cup water and ice.

MEAL 2: 1 cup steel cut oatmeal sprinkled with ground cinnamon and 1/2 cup fresh blueberries.

MEAL 3: Same as Meal 1.

MEAL 4: 8 ounces grilled chicken mixed with 1 cup brown rice, 1 tablespoon olive oil or salad dressing with 1 cup veggies.

MEAL 5: Myofusion Protein Pancakes: 1 scoop Myofusion, 1 cup egg whites, 1 cup oatmeal, 1/4 cup chopped walnuts, 1 sliced banana. Mix all together and cook on low heat on a non-stick pan using cooking spray. Optional: add sugar-free syrup.

MEAL 6: 8 ounces broiled mahi mahi or other white fish, 1 small potato, 3 ounces steamed string beans, 4 ounces green salad with vinegar.

MEAL 7 *(optional)*: Same as Meal 1.

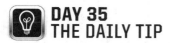 **DAY 35**
THE DAILY TIP

Remember the movie, Gremlins? Do you recall just how hungry those little critters got after midnight? Well, you have a similar beast within you, but it's a hormone—a Hungry Hormone called ghrelin. This little baby is responsible for skyrocketing our hunger senses and it's the predominant reason why we tend to overeat. Research has found that it can easily take a half-hour for the ghrelin to calm itself—way too long to wait for our brains to receive that fullness feeling. To combat the impact of ghrelin, try munching on a handful of almonds (about 100 calories' worth) 30 minutes before each meal. This will begin the digestion process and begin to get those messages translating from the belly to the brain.

DAY 36 BLAME IT ON THE HULK

As a young kid, I loved reading my older brother's comic books. *Captain America. Spider-Man. The Avengers. X-Men. The Fantastic Four. Superman. The Green Lantern. Batman. Wolverine.* They were all great. But when I got to a comic that featured *The Incredible Hulk,* he was instantly my favorite character. Scientist Robert Bruce Banner weighed only 130 pounds in the comic books—a lot more than I weighed at age nine—but when he turned into the Hulk he weighed close to 1,000 pounds! He was the strongest of all the comic book characters.

I'm still a little jealous that Lou Ferrigno, a great body-builder and friend, got to play Hulk in the CBS TV series that first aired when I was 16-years-old. Bill Bixby played Dr. David Banner—not sure why they changed his first name—and later directed some made-for-TV movies featuring the Hulk for NBC in the mid 80s. He and Lou reprised their roles. More recently, the Hulk has shown up in a couple of big screen movies as the Marvel franchise keeps churning out great entertainment, even if the movies and games are much more popular than the comic books themselves now.

There's a reason the appeal of comic book figures is powerful and enduring, especially for young boys. For many of us guys, they represented our first dreams about who we might become. We could get caught up in their fantasy world to escape whatever hardships we might be facing—or maybe simply to escape the boredom of everyday life. A superhero doesn't feel weak! So we were powerful, with super-human strengths—at least in our own minds. Sure, it's make-believe, but everyone knows a little make-believe is good for you.

Then, five or so years later, I saw my first bodybuilding magazine. My jaw dropped open. I couldn't believe what I was seeing. All I could think was, *unbelievable. There are comic book characters in real life. These guys look like they have superhuman powers. Look at them—I want to be like that.*

I never completely got away from the thought that I could actually train my body and look like the Hulk. I like to think I was better-looking and had better articulation than my green alter-ego. But he was my in-spiration from the world of fantasy.

People will tell you to grow up and get your head out of the clouds. It's true we need to grow in responsibility and character with every pass-ing year. We need to take care of business and look out for those people who matter most in our lives. But I hope I never grow to the point that I can't daydream about the Hulk and achieving superhuman accomplish-ments. When our ability to dream dies, so does our aspiration to be bet-ter than we are now. I may never get bigger physically than I am right now. But I hope Rich Gaspari, the businessman *and* the person, still has a lot more growing and dreaming to do.

So who do you want to be like *before* you grow up? As long as you're dreaming of being better, it's all good.

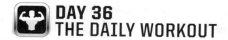 **DAY 36**
THE DAILY WORKOUT

THE MUSCLE BUILDER: CHEST & ABS
(Take 45 seconds - 1 minute rest between each set)
Incline dumbbell press – 4 sets of 8-10 reps
Incline dumbbell flies – 4 sets of 8-10 reps
Decline cable flies – 4 sets of 8-10 reps
Superset: Dumbbell flat bench, Pec Dec – 4 sets of 8-10 reps
Crunches – 4 sets of 25-30 reps
Leg raises – 4 sets of 25-30 reps

CARDIO
20-30 minutes interval cardio on treadmill

HARDGAINER WORKOUT: CHEST/BACK/BICEPS/TRICEPS/CORE
Modified Compound Superset #1 – *Take 45 seconds rest before moving on to the 2nd exercise*
Incline Dumbbell Press: 3 sets of 4-6 reps (45 Sec Rest)
Barbell Bent Over Row: 3 sets of 4-6 reps (1 min rest)
Modified Compound Superset #2 – *Take 45 seconds rest before moving on to the 2nd exercise*
Flat Dumbbell Bench Press: 3 sets of 6-8 reps (45 Sec Rest)
Chin-Ups: 3 sets of 6-8 reps (Strap on weight if you can)(1 min rest)
   Note: If you cannot perform the Chin-up, either have someone spot you by using your legs off their hands for leverage or have them spot-push you up by the waist.
Superset #3 – *No rest between exercises:*
Barbell Curls: 3 sets of 8-10 reps (No Rest)
Close Grip Dumbbell Bench Press (Triceps): 3 sets of 8-10 reps (1 min rest)
Superset #4 – *No rest between exercises:*
Dumbbell Hammer Curls: 3 sets of 10-12 reps (No Rest)
Triceps Pushdowns: 3 sets of 10-12 reps (1 min rest)

Superset #4 – *No rest between exercises*
Plank: 2 sets of 1 Minute Static Contraction [No Rest]
Bicycle Maneuver: 2 sets of 30 reps [1 min rest]

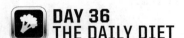

DAY 36
THE DAILY DIET

MEAL 1: Myofusion Shake: 2 scoops Myofusion, 1/2 cup egg whites, 2/3 cup instant oatmeal, 1 tablespoon natural peanut butter or almond butter, 1/2 cup apple juice, 1/2 cup water and ice.

MEAL 2: Myofusion Protein Pancakes: 1 scoop Myofusion, 1 cup egg whites, 1 cup oatmeal, 1/4 cup chopped walnuts, 1 sliced banana. Mix all together and cook on low heat on a non-stick pan using cooking spray. Optional: add sugar-free syrup.

MEAL 3: Same as Meal 1.

MEAL 4: 8 ounces grilled chicken breast, 1 cup quinoa, 1 cup steamed broccoli.

MEAL 5: 10 raw almonds.

MEAL 6: 8 ounces of lean steak, 1 sweet potato, 1 cup raw kale salad with 1 teaspoon olive oil and lemon juice.

MEAL 7 [*optional*]: Same as Meal 1.

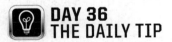

DAY 36
THE DAILY TIP

The key to the dumbbell chest press is to lower the weights beside your chest as far as possible. This completely stretches the pectorals before they are completely contracted at the height of the motion.

DAY 37 DO WHATEVER IT TAKES

My career in bodybuilding coincided almost perfectly with the journalism career of Lonnie Teper, probably the most prolific writer in the history of the sport. If you have ever attended a professional or NPC bodybuilding event, there's a good chance you've seen him live as he has hosted and emceed more than 250 events. He has a great background as a general sportswriter, sports editor, and even sports information director at a university. He's won a lot of awards for his writing and it's always a good time when he interviews me. One of the reasons is he has such an incredible memory. About a year ago, he interviewed me for *Iron Man* magazine and the first thing he said to me was, "Rich, I remember when you were getting started in your business career. You would show up at events and rent a six-foot table and two chairs. I can't believe how far you've come."

I've already shared how I was not prepared for the transition from professional athlete to the "real world." I had a couple years of college finished but had devoted all my energy to the sport I loved. I just assumed it would be easy to set up a successful gym and training business back home in New Jersey. Didn't happen that way. It only took me about a year to lose everything. But I fought back and determined I would do whatever it took to build a successful business.

In the early days, that meant renting the smallest, cheapest space available in the exhibit halls at bodybuilding events. I didn't have a fancy booth to set up. I had my own tablecloth to throw over the table and a small sign. I was usually in the back of the hall, so if I wanted business I couldn't sit on my butt and wait for people to come to me. I had to get out in the aisle and smile and shake hands and talk to as many people as I could in hopes they would take a look at my supplement products.

It was a humbling experience. I had gone from center stage with thousands cheering for me and the cameras capturing my every move to the back of the exhibit hall. I know some people felt sorry for me. I can't tell you how many times I heard things like, "Too bad about Rich. Look what he has to do."

Now I'm not going to lie to you and pretend that everything was sunshine and roses. But I can tell you in all honesty I never wasted a second feeling sorry for myself. I may have felt a little desperate at times, hustling to stay afloat, but I didn't look at this as some great catastrophe. It was honest work. It was something I owned. And I had every confidence that I was going to be a success. I knew myself. And I knew I was the very same person who a couple years earlier had succeeded on center stage.

Lonnie is an honest guy, too, and he admitted to me he wasn't sure at first if I was going to make it. It did come as quite a surprise to him how much I had studied nutrition from my earliest days. He remembered me as perhaps the greatest "worker" in the history of bodybuilding, but he didn't know the depth to which I had documented every exercise and every calorie and nutrition intake—and even how much I slept and how that impacted my performance.

I'm glad Lonnie reminded me of what some would call my "humble beginnings" as a businessman. I don't look back at that time with one scintilla of embarrassment. I'm proud of myself. I was ready and willing to do whatever it took to be successful. Maybe it's because I grew up in a home where Dad taught us the value of an honest day's work, but I look at the world a little differently. I'm proud to work. I'm ready to do whatever it takes. Still.

Whether you are in the gym or on the job, I hope you feel a sense of pride for the work you do. I hope you have and embrace the attitude of doing whatever it takes in all your endeavors. I can't promise you'll get rich. But I can promise you'll have success.

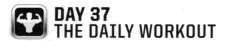

DAY 37
THE DAILY WORKOUT

THE MUSCLE BUILDER: BACK & CALVES
(Take 45 seconds - 1 minute rest between each set)

Deadlifts – 4 sets of 8-10 reps
Wide grip chins – 4 sets of 8-10 reps
Superset: Close grip pulldowns, Wide grip cable pullovers –
   4 sets of 8-10 reps
Superset: Cable low rows, T-bar rows – 4 sets of 8-10 reps
Superset: Two arm dumbbell rows, machine rows – 4 sets of 8-10 reps
Standing Calf raises – 5 sets of 15 reps
Seated calf raises – 5 sets of 15 reps

CARDIO
20-30 minutes interval cardio on treadmill

HARDGAINER WORKOUT:
THIGHS/HAMSTRINGS/DELTS/CALVES/LOWER ABS
Superset #1
Wide Stance Squats: 3 sets of 4-6 reps (45 Seconds Rest)
Stiff Legged Barbell Deadlifts: 3 sets of 4-6 reps (1 min rest)

> *Note: Utilize the "Full Body Tension Technique": This is when you
> stay in proper anatomical form and maintain that posture by
> keeping all of your major muscles contracted before & throughout
> the movements – This will keep you safe, while allowing you to use
> maximum intensity.*

Giant Set #2 – *3 exercises performed back-to-back without rest*
Leg Press: 3 sets of 6-8 reps (No Rest)
Leg Extensions: 3 sets of 10-12 reps (No Rest)
Lying Leg Curls: 3 sets of 10-12 reps (1 min rest)
Giant Set #3
Upright Barbell Row: 3 sets of 8-10 reps (No Rest)
Lateral Raises: 3 sets of 8-10 reps (No Rest)
Descending Set #4 – *Drop the weight as you move from set-to-set*

Standing Calf Raises (Gastrocs) - 3 Descending Sets – Decrease weight as you descend, if necessary:
  • 1st set of 12-15 reps (15 sec rest)
  • 2nd set of 12-15 reps (15 sec rest)
  • 3rd set of 12-15 reps (1 min rest & repeat 2 more times)

Superset #5

Bent Over Lateral Dumbbell Raises: 3 sets of 10-12 reps (No Rest)

Seated Calf Raises (Soleus): 3 sets of 10-12 reps (1 min rest)

Hanging Leg Raises: 3 sets of 15-20 reps (1 min rest)

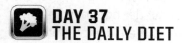 **DAY 37
THE DAILY DIET**

MEAL 1: Myofusion Shake: 2 scoops Myofusion, 1/2 cup egg whites, 2/3 cup instant oatmeal, 1 tablespoon natural peanut butter or almond butter, 1/2 cup apple juice, 1/2 cup water and ice.

MEAL 2: Myofusion Protein Pancakes: 1 scoop Myofusion, 1 cup egg whites, 1 cup oatmeal, 1/4 cup chopped walnuts, 1 sliced banana. Mix all together and cook on low heat on a non-stick pan using cooking spray. Optional: add sugar-free syrup.

MEAL 3: Same as Meal 1.

MEAL 4: 8 ounces grilled chicken breast, 1 sweet potato, 1 cup steamed broccoli.

MEAL 5: Same as Meal 1.

MEAL 6: 8 ounces baked salmon, 1 cup brown rice, 1 cup asparagus.

MEAL 7 *[optional]*: Same as Meal 1.

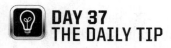 **DAY 37
THE DAILY TIP**

Today—challenge yourself. Set a goal of 50 deadlifts and do as many sets as it takes to hit that number.

DAY 38 NATURE VS. NURTURE

I like the old Eddie Murphy movie, *Trading Places*. His character starts out as a street hustler but ends up being a top commodity trader. He takes the place of a character played by Dan Akroyd who went to all the right schools but goes from the penthouse to the outhouse. How did these two guys get their lives turned upside down? Two billionaire brothers had a $1 bet on whether success was a matter of nature or nurture.

Nature or nurture? That particular debate will go on forever. And believe it or not, in the bodybuilding arena, it was a debate that included yours truly. That's right, the bodybuilding pundits were pretty convinced that I didn't have the genetics to be a champion. They said I was too small. Even when I did win, they said everything I accomplished was simply through sheer determination. Now that argument probably makes me look better than to say I was born with a freakish muscularity and had an easy climb to the top. The only problem is I don't think they are right.

Well . . . they were right about one thing. I wasn't born with Arnold's 6'2" frame. I wasn't born with Lee Haney's incredibly wide clavicles. Both Lee and Arnold were born with those tiny waists. I had to quit working abs before competitions because my waist was naturally thicker. So believe me, I know that genetics matter.

But let me ask you this. How many 140-pound teenagers can gain 40 pounds of muscle in one year? How many high schoolers are routinely working out with 450 pounds on the bench press and close to 700 pounds on squats? How many 48-year-olds can complete a 51-day workout transformation and get big and ripped enough to get back on the cover of *Iron Man* magazine—and look pretty darn good?

I'll also defend my genetics on the basis of my dad. He never worked out in a gym in his life, but he worked with brick and mortar all day. Even in his 50s and 60s and on into his retirement, he had a flat stomach and big muscular shoulders. He gave me my work ethic but he also passed on some pretty good genes for building muscle. I took what he gave me and made the most of it.

We all have strengths and weaknesses, and it's good to be honest about your own. But the truth about genetics is that it's only part of the equation. You definitely don't want to let whatever physical limitations you were born with make you want to give up or not work as hard as you should. Because nurture is just as important as nature. Fine tune your diet and workout program. Work harder to compensate for your areas of weakness. Work smarter and don't give up. Lee Haney was born with so much freakishness that he would have been a force in bodybuilding even if he hadn't been a hard worker. But the fact that he became training partners with a young dynamo named Rich Gaspari definitely contributed to his eight straight Mr. Olympia titles.

Maybe you weren't born with all the advantages others take for granted. Maybe your family was poor. Maybe you have a tendency to put on the wrong kind of weight. Maybe adding muscle and putting on weight is the hardest thing in the world for you. It doesn't matter. What matters is what you do with what you were born with. In building your ultimate body, you might need to add carbs or cut carbs. You might need to double your leg workout. You might need to add a longer aerobic period at the end of your workouts. The important thing is to understand what you've been given by nature and nurture it until you've reached your goals.

This isn't just a lesson for bodybuilding. If you tend to be shy but need to be more outgoing to get ahead in business, make yourself mingle. Read a book on conversation starters and get out there. Be thankful for your strengths and get to work on your weaknesses. That will count a lot more than being born with a high IQ and doing nothing with it. You might have a power chainsaw in the garage. It really isn't good for clearing snow off the driveway—but it's great for trimming tree limbs. It's worth nothing if it just sits there. You've been born with gifts. Nurture them and get moving!

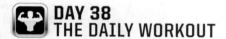

DAY 38
THE DAILY WORKOUT

THE MUSCLE BUILDER: LEGS
(Take 45 seconds - 1 minute rest between each set)
Lying leg curls – 5 sets of 10-12 reps
Stiff-legged deadlifts – 4 sets of 10-12 reps
Leg extensions – 5 sets of 10-12 reps (double drop set on last set)
45-degree Leg Press – 4 sets of 15 reps (double drop set on last set)
Hack Squat – 3 sets of 15 reps (triple drop set on last set)
Superset: Squats, walking lunges – 3 sets of 15-20 reps

CARDIO
20-30 minutes interval cardio on treadmill

HARDGAINER WORKOUT: REST

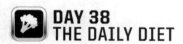

DAY 38
THE DAILY DIET

MEAL 1: Myofusion Shake: 2 scoops Myofusion, 1/2 cup egg whites, 2/3 cup instant oatmeal, 1 tablespoon natural peanut butter or almond butter, 1/2 cup apple juice, 1/2 cup water and ice.
MEAL 2: 8 ounces lean buffalo patty *(or 93% lean ground beef)* with salsa or mustard, 1 small potato, 6 ounces green salad with vinegar.
MEAL 3: Same as Meal 1.
MEAL 4: 8 ounces grilled chicken mixed with 1 cup brown rice, 1 tablespoon olive oil or salad dressing with 1 cup veggies.
MEAL 5: Same as Meal 1.
MEAL 6: Myofusion Protein Pancakes: 1 scoop Myofusion, 1 cup egg whites, 1 cup oatmeal, 1/4 cup chopped walnuts, 1 sliced banana. Mix all together and cook on low heat on a non-stick pan using cooking spray. Optional: add sugar-free syrup.
MEAL 7 *(optional)*: Same as Meal 1.

DAY 38
THE DAILY TIP

How is your energy and motivation in the gym? You might need a total change of pace. Jump into a basketball game or other running sport for your cardio. A spin class is a great cardio workout. Attend a yoga class for core and flexibility. Find a hardcore hiking trail. Play paintball with some fellow warriors. Do a ropes course. Swim laps. Find a change of pace activity and have a blast.

DAY 39 WHAT'S IN A NAME?

There is a story about the legendary Greek general, Alexander the Great, that I love. One of his soldiers kept getting in trouble with his commanding officers to the point that he was going to be executed. He was a drunk. He stole. He shirked his duties. Alexander heard that one of his men was to be executed and ordered that he be brought to his tent to see if he deserved mercy. First question he asked is, "What's your name?" The soldier answered, "Alexander." The man who conquered the known world was speechless for a minute as he let that sink in. He decided to give the man another chance but dismissed him with the command: "Change your name or change your ways."

What's your name? Oh I know you have a family name and a given name, but what about your nicknames? How do people perceive you?

Lonnie Teper was the first one to try a nickname on me. He called me Richie Ripped. It didn't stick. The nickname that did stick was "Dragon Slayer."

I think I actually appreciate that name more now than when I first got it. Jeff Everson, a well-known bodybuilder who went on to become a writer, wrote an article called "Rich Gaspari the Dragon Slayer."

The reason Jeff gave me that moniker was because I was often the smallest competitor in my class—but I knew how to cut the big guys down to size. I could take on the gargantuan competitors because of my superior conditioning. I introduced new levels of being ripped to the sport. I would say another advantage that allowed me to bring down bigger opponents than me was my mental toughness. I came to competitions so prepared that I just exuded confidence as I went about my business. I wasn't trying to psyche anyone out, but you'd better believe if an opponent came in even a little out of shape, he was already worried. And it showed.

Being known as the Dragon Slayer means a lot to me. It means I'm fearless in the face of adversity and danger. It means I have the character and nobility of a knight. It means I am willing to leave the comfort zone of my castle and make life an adventure. It means I'm willing to do what others flee from.

When I started this 51-day program, I wasn't out of shape. I didn't have a big gut. I wasn't showing up in business meetings and making appearances at competitions and having people look at me in shock and wondering, "What in the heck happened to Gaspari? When did he let himself go?" But I knew I had lost the edge that maximized my career—and really the same edge that had helped me make a success of my business—against much bigger competitors. I think I realized it was time to change my name or change my ways. No way was I going to give up being known as the Dragon Slayer—so it was time to change my ways and dig in.

If no one has given you a nickname you are crazy about, don't worry about it. Make up your own nickname. You don't even have to tell anyone. It can be your own secret. But once you do that, then it's time to live up to the name you give yourself. You either have to change your name or change your ways. Earn that name with your absolute best workout so far today!

DAY 39
THE DAILY WORKOUT

THE MUSCLE BUILDER: SHOULDERS & ABS
[Take 45 seconds - 1 minute rest between each set]
Seated barbell front press – 4 sets of 8-12 reps
Giantset: Seated side laterals, Arnold Press, Standing dumbbell upright
   rows – 4 sets of 10-12 reps
Incline one arm side laterals – 3 sets of 12-15
Machine rear laterals – 4 sets of 12-15
Barbell shrugs from behind – 4 sets of 12-15
Twisting crunches – 4 sets of 30 reps
Leg raises – 4 sets of 25 reps

CARDIO
20-30 minutes interval cardio on treadmill

HARDGAINER WORKOUT: CHEST/BACK/BICEPS/TRICEPS/ABS
Modified Compound Superset #1
Flat Dumbbell Bench Press: 3 sets of 8, 6, 4 reps [90 second rest]
Close Grip Neutral Grip Pull-Ups: 3 sets of 8, 6, 4 reps
   [Strap weight on if you can – 2 mins rest]
   *Note: If you cannot perform the Close Grip Pull-Up, either have
   someone spot you by using your legs off their hands for leverage
   or have them spot-push you up by the waist.*
Modified Compound Superset #2
Incline Barbell Bench Press: 3 sets of 8, 6, 4 reps [90 second rest]
Bent Over Underhand Barbell Row: 3 sets of 8, 6, 4 reps [2 min rest]
Giant Modified Compound Super Set #3 – *Take prescribed rest
   between exercise*
Chest Dips: 3 sets of 8, 6, 4 reps [60 second rest]
Preacher Curls: 3 sets of 8, 6, 4 reps [45 second rest]
Close Grip Bench Press: 3 sets of 8, 6, 4 reps [2 min rest]
Giant Modified Compound Super Set #4
E-Z Preacher Curls: 3 sets of 8, 6, 4 reps [60 second rest]

Lying Triceps Extensions: 3 sets of 8, 6, 4 reps (45 second rest)
Swiss Ball (aka "Inflated Fitness Ball") Crunches: 3 sets of 20, 15, 10 reps (Hold a weight plate or dumbbell overhead if you can) (2 min rest)

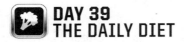

DAY 39
THE DAILY DIET

MEAL 1: Myofusion Shake: 2 scoops Myofusion, 1/2 cup egg whites, 2/3 cup instant oatmeal, 1 tablespoon natural peanut butter or almond butter, 1/2 cup apple juice, 1/2 cup water and ice.

MEAL 2: Myofusion Protein Pancakes: 1 scoop Myofusion, 1 cup egg whites, 1 cup oatmeal, 1/4 cup chopped walnuts, 1 sliced banana. Mix all together and cook on low heat on a non-stick pan using cooking spray. Optional: add sugar-free syrup.

MEAL 3: 10 raw almonds.

MEAL 4: 8 ounces grilled chicken, 1 cup quinoa, 1 cup grilled squash and zucchini drizzled with balsamic vinegar and 1 tablespoon olive oil.

MEAL 5: Same as Meal 1.

MEAL 6: Egg omelet: 1 cup egg whites mixed with 1 cup chopped peppers, onions, and tomatoes. 1 slice watermelon on the side.

MEAL 7 *(optional)*: Same as Meal 1.

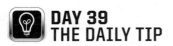

DAY 39
THE DAILY TIP

Procrastination often leads to regret. I don't know about you, but I cannot stand those times when I've said to myself, "I should've done this or that." For me personally, I've never been okay with the "should haves" or "could haves." Why? Because it's never too late to jump in! You can make up for lost time by starting over right now!

DAY 40 NEVER STOP LEARNING

When I first got into bodybuilding, I was like a sponge. I soaked up everything I could learn. I watched. I listened. I scribbled notes in a journal. I read everything I could get my hands on. There weren't many books on bodybuilding, but I saved up my nickels and dimes from a paper route and bought them all. I subscribed to all the magazines and read them from cover to cover. I bought anything that had to do with improving performance. I learned a lot on my own. But whether it was seeing what others were doing in the gym or magazine interviews, I took it all in!

When I overcame some early setbacks, bad decisions, and bad plans and finally got my company going, I don't think it was a coincidence that I had also rediscovered my passion for learning. I was a sponge again. I read Jim Collins' classic business book, *Good to Great*. I read Steven Covey's *7 Habits of Highly Successful People*. I read Dale Carnegie's *How to Win Friends and Influence People*. I read W. Chan Kim and Renee Maubornge's *Blue Ocean Strategy*. I started subscribing to the *Wall Street Journal* every day. I'll tell you, it wasn't easy to switch from glossy magazines with lots of pictures talking about the thing I liked most—bodybuilding—and make myself learn to compete in a whole new arena. But I picked up how-to manuals on writing a business plan, setting up an accounting system, hiring the right people, managing people, getting a line of credit, effective marketing, how to be a great sales person, and more. It took a great team for Gaspari Nutrition to become such a success.

I think one of the most dangerous things anyone of us can ever say is, "I already know how to do that." It may be true to some extent. You may be very knowledgable and experienced. But things change—technology, markets, consumer tastes and needs, and so much more. Even if there was no change and life was static, even if we were convinced we were the best and the brightest in our area of interests, I'll bet you and I both know less than we think we do.

Learning is for a lifetime. I think that's the biggest lesson I learned from my rough transition from being a competitor to building a career. I thought I could do it all with reputation, enthusiasm, and hustle. Those things helped—and they kept me going when times were tough, but when I started hitting the books again I realized how much more I needed to know if I was going to get ahead. And you know what—it wasn't just the specific things I learned that helped so much. It was the attitude of wanting to learn that made such a huge difference.

Life is not a destination—it's a journey. You've heard that. And that is what I mean by becoming a sponge. It's not *what* you learn—it's simply about always learning. An active, never ending process.

I may have never met you personally, but I already respect you. Why? You bought a book. You thought, *I need to know what Rich Gaspari can tell me to improve my performance and achieve a better body*. Eighty percent of Americans don't even buy or read one book per year. You've already put yourself in the top 20%. Don't stop now. Mark Twain got it right when he said, "A person who *won't* read has no advantage over one who *can't* read." Don't stop with this program and your body. Don't make the same mistake I made by not reading when I needed to the most. Start now. Everything changes when you make the commitment to never stop learning.

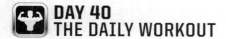

DAY 40
THE DAILY WORKOUT

THE MUSCLE BUILDER: BICEPS & TRICEPS
(Take 45 seconds - 1 minute rest between each set)
Superset: Incline dumbbell curls, Rope pushdowns – 4 sets of 10 reps
Superset: Standing barbell curls, Seated 2-arm overhead tricep
extension with Dumbbell – 4 sets of 10 reps
Superset: Seated preacher curls with EZ curl bar,
Lying pullover press – 4 sets of 10 reps
Superset: Dumbbell concentration curls, cable kickbacks
– 4 sets of 10 reps

CARDIO
20-30 minutes interval cardio on treadmill

HARDGAINER WORKOUT: THIGHS/HAMSTRINGS/DELTS/CALVES
Modified Compound Superset #1
Medium Stance Squats: 3 sets of 8, 6, 4 reps (90 second rest)
Lying Leg Curls: 3 sets of 8, 6, 4 reps (90 second rest)
> *Note: If you suffer from lower back problems you may substitute the
> squat for the leg press. Since you are performing the leg press as
> your second exercise, then just use a close stance on this one and
> a medium stance on the second one.*

Modified Compound Superset #2
Leg Press: 3 sets of 8, 6, 4 reps (90 second rest)
Barbell Romanian Deadlifts: 3 sets of 8, 6, 4 reps (2 min rest)
Modified Compound Superset #3
Seated Barbell Front Shoulder: 3 sets of 8, 6, 4 reps (60 second rest)
Standing Calf Raise (Gastrocs): 3 sets of 10, 8, 6 reps (2 min rest)
Modified Compound Superset #4
Dumbbell Lateral Raises: 3 sets of 8, 6, 4 reps (60 second rest)
Lying Leg Raises with a pop at the top of each rep: 3 sets of 10, 8, 6
reps (60 second rest)
Descending Set #5 – *Drop the weight as you move from set-to-set*

Seated Calf Raises (Soleus) - 3 Descending Sets – Decrease weight as you descend, if necessary:
- 1st set of 12-15 reps (15 sec rest)
- 2nd set of 12-15 reps (15 sec rest)
- 3rd set of 12-15 reps (1 min rest & repeat 2 more times)

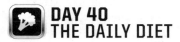 **DAY 40**
THE DAILY DIET

MEAL 1: Myofusion Shake: 2 scoops Myofusion, 1/2 cup egg whites, 2/3 cup instant oatmeal, 1 tablespoon natural peanut butter or almond butter, 1/2 cup apple juice, 1/2 cup water and ice.

MEAL 2: 1 cup steel cut oatmeal sprinkled with ground cinnamon and 1/2 cup fresh blueberries.

MEAL 3: Same as Meal 1.

MEAL 4: 8 ounces grilled chicken breast, 1 cup brown rice, 1 cup steamed broccoli.

MEAL 5: Same as Meal 1.

MEAL 6: 8 ounces of lean steak, 1 sweet potato, 1/2 cup mushrooms, 6 ounces green salad with vinegar.

MEAL 7 [optional]: Same as Meal 1.

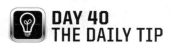 **DAY 40**
THE DAILY TIP

A cup of coffee before a workout? Caffeine happens to be a great ergogenic training aid and a fuel that provides quick energy and gets your blood pumping. When you ingest caffeine before a workout, just be careful to drink lots of water, as the excess caffeine can dehydrate you. In fact, you should always make sure to sip water before, during, and after your workouts in order to stay hydrated.

DAY 41 FAMILY PRIDE

The story of my dad's journey from Italy to America could easily be a stand-alone book. It is one of those adventures that usually leads people to say, "Truth is stranger than fiction." My dad was traditional and conservative and he loved his native Italy. But from a very early age, he wanted to come to America. He believed in the promise of the American dream—that America truly was a land of opportunity. He definitely passed that belief on to me, so I come by it honestly. He admitted he may have been a little naive when he believed stories he heard that the streets were paved with gold. But when he finally got to the U.S. and built a life for his family, he never had second thoughts about his decision to get here. He was never disappointed.

A big reason my dad came to America is because he believed in work—it drove him crazy how many of his friends in Italy spent the day in the town square smoking cigarettes and drinking coffee all day. When I visited Italy about a decade ago there were still people alive who remembered my dad. I got a good laugh and felt a lot of pride when I was told numerous times, "He worked too hard, he had too much ambition to stay here."

A number of my uncles arrived in the United States before the start of World War II—and one of them went back to Europe to fight with the U.S. Army. But my dad was the youngest and was the only one still living in the family's hometown when my granddad died, so he had to stay and support his mom. That's when he first became a stonemason.

Once the war started, it became impossible for him to leave. He was drafted into the Italian army and spent most of the war in what was then Yugoslavia. I've never heard him talk about politics much, but I do know that growing up he felt the greatest threat to world security was Communism, which makes sense due to his time in Eastern Europe.

Italy had some grandiose notions under Mussolini and one of his plans was to take over large sections of Africa and make them Italian colonies. Sounds crazy now, but Mussolini felt like Italians could teach locals to cultivate the land and create not only a large bread basket, but also develop some great wine regions. I love my glass of red wine and that's something else I came by honestly with my Italian background. My dad was put on an advance landing ship that was torpedoed by the British. A couple thousand men died, but my dad survived and finished the war as a POW.

Because my dad fought in the Italian army, he couldn't come straight to America after the war, but he was still determined to get here. There were more opportunities for him at the time in Australia and South America, but he picked Canada—it was closer to his real goal. It would be easier to get to the U.S. from there.

So he and my mom landed in Canada with two sons and a daughter. They arrived in the middle of winter. He swears there was twenty feet of snow piled everywhere. All he had was a thin jacket. He would joke that he left the warm, temperate Mediterranean region and landed in a "frozen hell." Another brother was born in Canada and it took my parents 10 years to complete the move to New Jersey. I was their only child born in the U.S.

My dad never got rich in this land of opportunity, but he always had a job and was able to provide for us. I think one of the great things about that era was the amount of pride people had in being everyday blue-collar workers. Now people look down on being a "common worker." I can't stand it when I hear journalists and commentators talk disparagingly about what they describe as "menial" work. Work is work. It's all good. We all need to take more pride in showing up for a job, paying our bills, and putting food on the table.

I love my family history. My parents didn't have an easy journey. But what they taught me was the power of determination. They taught me to believe in the American Dream, too. I know the economy has taken some hits. There's a business cycle that has some peaks and valleys and we've been in the valley for a while. Too many people are out of work and I know for many of them it's not because they are lazy or don't want to work. But before you complain about a job being too hard, it might be good to remember that it beats the alternative of no work.

Hard work. Determination. Seizing opportunities. That's what my family's journey from Italy to america taught me.

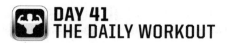

DAY 41
THE DAILY WORKOUT

THE MUSCLE BUILDER: REST

HARDGAINER WORKOUT: REST

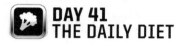

DAY 41
THE DAILY DIET

MEAL 1: Myofusion Shake: 2 scoops Myofusion, 1/2 cup egg whites, 2/3 cup instant oatmeal, 1 tablespoon natural peanut butter or almond butter, 1/2 cup apple juice, 1/2 cup water and ice.

MEAL 2: Myofusion Protein Pancakes: 1 scoop Myofusion, 1 cup egg whites, 1 cup oatmeal, 1/4 cup chopped walnuts, 1 sliced banana. Mix all together and cook on low heat on a non-stick pan using cooking spray. Optional: add sugar-free syrup.

MEAL 3: Same as Meal 1.

MEAL 4: Egg omelet: 1 cup egg whites mixed with 1 cup chopped peppers, onions, and tomatoes. 1 slice watermelon on the side.

MEAL 5: 10 raw almonds.

MEAL 6: 8 ounces mahi mahi or other white fish, 1 small potato, 3 ounces steamed string beans, 4 ounces green salad with vinegar.

MEAL 7 [optional]**:** Same as Meal 1.

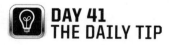

DAY 41
THE DAILY TIP

What you are today is a product of what you did yesterday. What you are tomorrow is a product of what you do today.

DAY 42 ONE PENNY AT A TIME

One of the things that drives me crazy in my industry is the number of diet products that are marketed as a quick fix to a long-term problem. I'm amazed at how many people will sit back and let themselves go, but suddenly start to worry about what their body looks like because of some event that is coming up. *My friend is getting married and I want to look good in a sleeveless dress. My 20th class reunion is coming up and I don't want anyone to see how much weight I've gained over the years.* The classic is, *"We're going to the beach this summer and no way do I want to put on a swimsuit looking the way I do now."*

Now I'm sympathetic to a degree. I understand circumstances come up. Everyone goes through challenging seasons in life. If you're working a full time job and taking night classes, you might not have as much time to look your best. If you sprain an ankle playing some basketball or tennis, you are going to lose workout time. Heck, I've torn muscles and done ligament damage, so I know there are times when an aggressive workout schedule just isn't possible. But too many people take way too much time off or fall into all kinds of bad habits and then get frustrated when they lose their physique.

One of the things that worries me about people taking a feast or famine approach to their workouts is that when they get back on track, they start to get impatient and try some stupid stuff with their diet, supplementation, and workout routine hoping to get in shape in a hurry. The bot-

196 | RICH GASPARI

tom line is that getting the body you want isn't a quick fix program—it's really not just 51 days. It's a lifestyle. It takes consistent planning and work to eat right, add the right supplements, and stay with a hard work-out program.

We know this is part of life. The tortoise beats the hare. The diligent ant eats when the lazy grasshopper starves. The farmer doesn't take one spring off from planting and expect a harvest that fall. The shop owner doesn't decide to take off the months of November and December when his store is busiest and expect that he can save his business with a good January, the worst shopping month of the year.

I can guarantee you I would not have won as many championships as I did if some of my competitors had been more diligent and consistent. There were some genetic marvels who just didn't stay the course. Even when a competition was coming up they would take days off from their regime. Bodybuilding contests don't work that way and neither does life.

But I need some down time. There's plenty of rest time in any good bodybuilding workout program. You get two to three days off per week depending on which program you follow with me.

The dieting is hard for me. I would encourage you to not take time off from the diet, even for the holidays. There are a lot of healthy recipes to give you the variety of foods you want. It may take you awhile to get in the rhythm, but once you do, you'll be eating six or seven times a day. That doesn't sound like a tough diet to me.

Supplements and specialty foods are more expensive. If I could buy what I needed at age 14 and 15 with nothing but a paper route, I know you can find a way too. We spend our money on what's important to us. What could be more important than your body?

What you may most need to do is change your mindset. Do you *have* to go the gym tomorrow? Or do you *get* to go the gym tomorrow? Some of us have been conditioned to dread things that are hard. Why not look at things differently and see that tough superset I have outlined for you as a fun dare and challenge rather than something unpleasant?

When I was a kid I had a piggy bank. No one gave me a bunch of money to add to it, so I had to watch it grow one penny, nickel, and dime at a time. Guess what? That's the same way we build and maintain an ultimate body. One penny at a time.

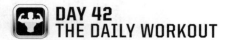

DAY 42
THE DAILY WORKOUT

THE MUSCLE BUILDER: REST

HARDGAINER WORKOUT: REST

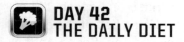

DAY 42
THE DAILY DIET

MEAL 1: Myofusion Shake: 2 scoops Myofusion, 1/2 cup egg whites, 2/3 cup instant oatmeal, 1 tablespoon natural peanut butter or almond butter, 1/2 cup apple juice, 1/2 cup water and ice.

MEAL 2: Myofusion Protein Pancakes: 1 scoop Myofusion, 1 cup egg whites, 1 cup oatmeal, 1/4 cup chopped walnuts, 1 sliced banana. Mix all together and cook on low heat on a non-stick pan using cooking spray. Optional: add sugar-free syrup.

MEAL 3: Same as Meal 1.

MEAL 4: 8 ounces grilled chicken, 1 cup brown rice, 1 apple.

MEAL 5: Same as Meal 1.

MEAL 6: 8 ounces lean ground beef, 1 cup gluten-free pasta, 4-6 ounces low sodium natural tomato sauce with 1 tablespoon grated cheese *(optional)*.

MEAL 7 *(optional)*: Same as Meal 1.

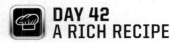

DAY 42
A RICH RECIPE

CHOCOLATE-COVERED STRAWBERRY MYOFUSION PARFAIT
A Healthy and Sweet Treat from Jaime Baird

1/2 scoop MyoFusion Chocolate protein

1/2 scoop MyoFusion Strawberries & Cream protein

6 ounces plain, nonfat Greek yogurt

2 large strawberries

1 chocolate wafer, less than 40 calories

1/3 ounce semi-sweet chocolate

In a small bowl, mix the MyoFusion and Greek yogurt until completely blended. Place bowl in refrigerator. Slice one strawberry and set aside. Place the chocolate wafer in a ziplock bag and crush it into small crumbs.

Remove MyoFusion yogurt mixture from fridge and spoon 1/2 of mixture into a serving glass or bowl. Then sprinkle on half of the cookie crumbs and place half of the strawberry slices on top. Spoon on the remainder of the MyoFusion yogurt mixture. Layer the remaining cookie crumbs and strawberry slices on top.

Microwave 1/3 ounce semi-sweet chocolate in a glass bowl for 30 seconds. Stir and continue microwaving at 10-second intervals until chocolate is completely melted. Dip a strawberry into the melted chocolate and swirl until it is completely coated. Place strawberry on wax paper and refrigerate for 20 min. When ready to serve, remove strawberry from the refrigerator and use as a garnish for the parfait. Makes 1 serving.

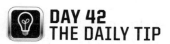 DAY 42
THE DAILY TIP

Leaving your comfort zone is the key to progress. This applies not only to your workouts, but also the gym as well. Every now and then it's a good idea to switch gyms, even if it's just for a one day pass. This is a great way to experiment with new equipment and reinvigorate yourself.

DAY 43 THIS IS WAR

Here's a little secret you may not be aware of. The human body does not want to become big and muscular. We have evolved over hundreds of thousands of years from hunter-gatherers whose survival depended on being able to move to where the food was, hunt or gather the food, and also to be able to subsist for long periods without food. There were no supermarkets, or even farms, back in the Ice Age. Having a lot of muscle mass would have been a handicap, believe it or not. All that muscle takes a lot of calories and protein to feed, after all. Our bodies would much prefer to stay smaller and thus require less effort to maintain.

What does that mean to you as a bodybuilder or an aspiring bodybuilder? Simply put, you are literally at war with your own body in your quest. How do you win this war? You push your muscles harder than they have ever been pushed before! It's this "shock" that forces your muscles to adapt by growing bigger and stronger. This is why it takes real effort to build mass, not just messing around with weights.

It also means it takes greater effort and intensity as the months and years go by to stimulate more gains. Few people are willing to keep "raising the bar" by forcing themselves to use more weight. They can't push themselves past the pain barrier and get in one more rep than last time, over and over again. That's why most guys in the gym reach a certain level and never get past that. You see them all the time, and they always look exactly the same.

I know you don't want to be one of them!

Slinging around weight will not produce the results you are looking for. I always use strict form and a controlled rep speed. I pause at the completion of each rep and squeeze the muscle for all it's worth, then fight the negative so the muscle gets a good stretch on the way down. There are no half-reps. Using a full range of motion is the best way to fully develop the muscle. And when you train, that's how you need to think of it—training the muscle. I seek out a deep burn inside the belly of the muscle by getting about eight reps into a set. Getting a full-blown pump is the goal, but the real challenge is being able to do that with heavy weights. Anybody off the street can take a light weight, do fifty reps of curls with it, and his biceps will get pumped. It takes a strong mind-muscle connection to generate that same feeling with a weight you can only get for seven or eight reps.

I'm sure you've heard the cliché, "When the going gets tough, the tough get going." Cliché or not, this is the ideal that I live by. I've told you before that when things get tough on the gym floor, I'm just getting started. In my mind, every workout is do or die. Doing things half-assed isn't going to work. You need to train like a soldier in boot camp. You need to steel yourself against the pain and determine to push beyond your limitations. You are in a war—you against your body. Are you ready to fight? Are you ready to win?

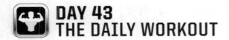 **DAY 43**
THE DAILY WORKOUT

THE MUSCLE BUILDER: CHEST & ABS
(Take 45 seconds - 1 minute rest between each set)
Incline dumbbell press – 4 sets of 8-10 reps
Incline dumbbell flies – 4 sets of 8-10 reps
Decline cable flies – 4 sets of 8-10 reps
Superset: Dumbbell flat bench, Pec Dec – 4 sets of 8-10 reps
Crunches – 4 sets of 25-30 reps
Leg raises – 4 sets of 25-30 reps

CARDIO
20-30 minutes interval cardio on treadmill

HARDGAINER WORKOUT: CHEST/BACK/BICEPS/TRICEPS/CORE
Modified Compound Superset #1 – *Take 45 seconds rest before moving on to the 2nd exercise*
Incline Dumbbell Press: 3 sets of 4-6 reps (45 Sec Rest)
Barbell Bent Over Row: 3 sets of 4-6 reps (1 min rest)
Modified Compound Superset #2 – *Take 45 seconds rest before moving on to the 2nd exercise*
Flat Dumbbell Bench Press: 3 sets of 6-8 reps (45 Sec Rest)
Chin-Ups: 3 sets of 6-8 reps (Strap on weight if you can)(1 min rest)
  Note: If you cannot perform the Chin-up, either have someone spot you by using your legs off their hands for leverage or have them spot-push you up by the waist.
Superset #3 – *No rest between exercises*
Barbell Curls: 3 sets of 8-10 reps (No Rest)
Close Grip Dumbbell Bench Press (Triceps): 3 sets of 8-10 reps (1 min rest)
Superset #4 – *No rest between exercises*
Dumbbell Hammer Curls: 3 sets of 10-12 reps (No Rest)
Triceps Pushdowns: 3 sets of 10-12 reps (1 min rest)
Superset #5 – *No rest between exercises*

Plank: 2 sets of 1 Minute Static Contraction (No Rest)
Bicycle Maneuver: 2 sets of 30 reps (1 min rest)

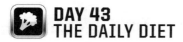

DAY 43
THE DAILY DIET

MEAL 1: Myofusion Shake: 2 scoops Myofusion, 1/2 cup egg whites, 2/3 cup instant oatmeal, 1 tablespoon natural peanut butter or almond butter, 1/2 cup apple juice, 1/2 cup water and ice.

MEAL 2: Myofusion Protein Pancakes: 1 scoop Myofusion, 1 cup egg whites, 1 cup oatmeal, 1/4 cup chopped walnuts, 1 sliced banana. Mix all together and cook on low heat on a non-stick pan using cooking spray. Optional: add sugar-free syrup.

MEAL 3: 10 raw almonds.

MEAL 4: 8 ounces grilled chicken, 1 cup quinoa, 6 ounces green salad with vinegar.

MEAL 5: Same as Meal 1.

MEAL 6: 8 ounces grilled tuna, 1 cup brown rice, 1 teaspoon of olive oil, 1 cup asparagus.

MEAL 7 [optional]**:** Same as Meal 1.

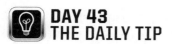

DAY 43
THE DAILY TIP

The use of probiotics not only aids the health of your immune system, but also increases the utilization of protein supplements by improving digestion, leading to better gains.

DAY 44 FORGE YOUR OWN PATH

I've encouraged you throughout this book to make a point of learning everything you can. None of us has all the answers. We can benefit from the experiences of others in so many ways. We can get in better shape, become a more valuable worker, gain promotions, and we can also improve our marriage or our parenting skills. I've learned a lot through the years and I love sharing the wisdom and insights I've gained in my own life. But sometimes the hard thing is knowing when to stop listening to all of the advice that well-meaning friends, family, and even "experts" want to give you and figure out what works best for *you*.

When I started my 51-day transformation, I started seeing my body change in ways I hadn't seen in more than fifteen years! Seeing my body get leaner and leaner and seeing muscle detail that I hadn't seen in so long really fueled my motivation to stay on my diet and continue to make gains I thought wouldn't come back due to my age or the many injuries I had sustained throughout the years. On the contrary, it seemed once I got in the groove with my training and my eating, I saw changes happening more easily than I thought.

One thing I had assumed was that I would have to do a high volume of cardio to get to my ripped condition of the late 80s and 90s. So when I began, I did 30 minutes of sprints and fast walking to help start the leaning-out process. What I quickly noticed after a week of adding in

204 | RICH GASPARI

cardio was that with dieting strictly and weight training hard and consistently, I was losing weight too quickly. I had a choice of either trying to eat even more or cut out cardio completely, and watch to see if my body would change. I chose to keep my diet the same and stop the cardio. As long as I saw that I was getting leaner, I didn't do any cardio at all.

This is just an example of being able to monitor your body effectively, and not giving in to the pressure of doing what other people say you "have" to do. I see it all the time with today's professional bodybuilders needing a trainer to tell them how to train, how much cardio to do, or how much to eat. They would rather leave all that up to someone else and basically hand over the keys!

This is something I believe every individual has to be able to figure out for him or herself. Everyone is different when it comes to dieting and training. Dieting is often a process of trial and error, so you can learn what works for you. There are some big name trainers and coaches who follow the same diet concept for all their clients; only to have success with some of them and failure with others. It's ridiculous to think everyone can eat exactly the same way and get into great condition.

This book is all about sharing the secrets and lessons I've learned in my life and career, and especially on my 51-day journey. I hope that you have been inspired and have gained new information that helps you succeed and stay motivated to achieve your ultimate body. But guess what? Sometimes you may need to say, "Hey Rich, thanks for the advice, but I'm going to try doing things a little differently. I'm not getting the same results as you and I have a couple ideas I want to try."

You won't offend me. In fact, I take my hat off to you. You're taking initiative. You're owning your own version of a 51-day ultimate body program. Even if what you try doesn't work, you won't hear me telling you, "I told you so." We learn from others. But we also have to forge our own path.

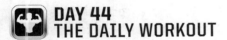

DAY 44
THE DAILY WORKOUT

THE MUSCLE BUILDER: BACK & CALVES
[Take 45 seconds - 1 minute rest between each set]

Deadlifts – 4 sets of 8-10 reps
Wide grip chins – 4 sets of 8-10 reps
Superset: Close grip pulldowns, Wide grip cable pullovers – 4 sets of 8-10 reps
Superset: Cable low rows, T-bar rows – 4 sets of 8-10 reps
Superset: Two arm dumbbell rows, machine rows – 4 sets of 8-10 reps
Standing Calf raises – 5 sets of 15 reps
Seated calf raises – 5 sets of 15 reps

CARDIO
20-30 minutes interval cardio on treadmill

HARDGAINER WORKOUT:
THIGHS/HAMSTRINGS/DELTS/CALVES/LOWER ABS
Superset #1
Wide Stance Squats: 3 sets of 4-6 reps [45 Seconds Rest]
Stiff Legged Barbell Deadlifts: 3 sets of 4-6 reps [1 min rest]

> *Note: Utilize the "Full Body Tension Technique": This is when you stay in proper anatomical form and maintain that posture by keeping all of your major muscles contracted before & throughout the movements – This will keep you safe, while allowing you to use maximum intensity.*

Giant Set #2 – *3 exercises performed back-to-back without rest*
Leg Press: 3 sets of 6-8 reps [No Rest]
Leg Extensions: 3 sets of 10-12 reps [No Rest]
Lying Leg Curls: 3 sets of 10-12 reps [1 min rest]
Giant Set #3
Upright Barbell Row: 3 sets of 8-10 reps [No Rest]
Lateral Raises: 3 sets of 8-10 reps [No Rest]

Descending Set #4 – *Drop the weight as you move from set–to–set*
Standing Calf Raises (Gastrocs) - 3 Descending Sets – Decrease
    weight as you descend, if necessary:
    • 1st set of 12-15 reps (15 sec rest)
    • 2nd set of 12-15 reps (15 sec rest)
    • 3rd set of 12-15 reps (1 min rest & repeat 2 more times)
Superset #5
Bent Over Lateral Dumbbell Raises: 3 sets of 10-12 reps (No Rest)
Seated Calf Raises (Soleus): 3 sets of 10-12 reps (1 min rest)
Hanging Leg Raises: 3 sets of 15-20 reps (1 min rest)

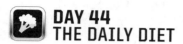

DAY 44
THE DAILY DIET

MEAL 1: Myofusion Shake: 2 scoops Myofusion, 1/2 cup egg whites,
    2/3 cup instant oatmeal, 1 tablespoon natural peanut butter
    or almond butter, 1/2 cup apple juice, 1/2 cup water and ice.
MEAL 2: 1 cup steel cut oatmeal sprinkled with ground cinnamon and
    1/2 cup fresh blueberries.
MEAL 3: Same as Meal 1.
MEAL 4: 8 ounces grilled chicken breast, 1 sweet potato, 1 cup grilled
    squash and zucchini drizzled with balsamic vinegar and 1
    tablespoon olive oil.
MEAL 5: Same as Meal 1.
MEAL 6: 8 ounces of lean steak, 1 cup quinoa, 1 cup raw kale salad with
    1 teaspoon olive oil and lemon juice.
MEAL 7 *(optional)*: Same as Meal 1.

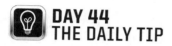

DAY 44
THE DAILY TIP

*A great way to start a back workout is a compound movement like the
bent over barbell row. Increase the weight but maintain great form, even
if you do fewer reps each time.*

DAY 45 THE WELL-ROUNDED CHEST

I want this book to focus on motivation, but let's be honest, probably nothing motivates guys or girls more than to have a great chest. The problem is I see more training mistakes on the chest than any other body area. Many beginners think the best way to get a great chest is to be a great bench presser. That is far from the truth if your goal is to have a well developed, all-around great chest.

In the beginning, the first thing I did was concentrate on getting my bench up. I felt that with a great bench, I would have an Arnold chest for sure! As I started to learn more, I found it took different exercises to really get a well-rounded chest. That meant great proportional development of the lower to upper chest, as well as having the inner and outer chest developed proportionally too. A chest like that is truly impressive to behold. What I have seen even with myself in my younger years is that doing just a lot of bench presses causes you to develop the "Droopy Chest Syndrome." This is a chest that has way too much development in the lower part, and not enough in the upper region. It almost looks like you've developed breasts! A great chest does not look like it needs a support bra, it's one that looks like a Roman Centurian's chest plate.

It all comes down to working out right, not just training hard with no strategy. Besides doing a variety of exercises to develop a well rounded chest, it's equally important to do the exercises properly. Doing the exercises with proper form will not only allow you to stress the target muscle fibers to the max, it will also help you prevent the various injuries that are all too easy to fall prey to if you are careless.

The most important form tip to keep in mind with any chest exercise is to stick your chest out by pinching your shoulder blades together before starting the set. This makes your pecs stick out past your shoulders so they won't be able to take over. What so many people do is throw their shoulder forward, making them hit less chest and more front delts. This is probably the one form error that keeps most guys from ever building a great chest.

Once you have that part of the form down, think about each rep as squeezing and stretching your pecs. This ensures a nice contraction and a good stretch, both of which are vital components to stimulating the muscle fibers of the chest and spurring growth. It takes practice, and you will have to use lighter weights to get the right form and feeling in the muscle down pat. But practice makes perfect, and in this case perfect practice is what will ultimately give you the perfectly developed chest you want.

Variety is also key, as you need to work the chest from various angles. A well developed chest requires you do compound or multi-joint mass building movements along with isolation movements. This means doing some form of pressing motion as well as doing some form of flye movement.

As I said earlier, the chest seems to develop easier in the lower part more than the upper part of the overall pecs when doing more flat bench or flat flye movements, so I have always concentrated on the upper chest first to get that well-balanced look. Some movements of the upper chest are exercises on an incline bench, which I do more on a 60-degree angle as opposed to a 45-degree angle like most people do. For me, the higher incline seems to hit my upper chest better.

Another great movement for upper development, believe it or not, is the reverse grip bench press. Research has actually shown that doing a reverse grip bench press recruited more upper chest than flat bench. It also gives you a totally different feel, so give it a try.

There are also advanced techniques in developing the chest that I have found deliver excellent results. One advanced technique is pre-exhaust, where you do an Isolation exercise like a flye supersetted with a compound movement like a bench press or incline press. In doing this, the isolation exercise fatigues the stronger chest muscle before the smaller triceps and shoulders fatigue, allowing you to train the chest to total failure. Too many people have problems where their triceps or front delts seem to fatigue first, giving those body parts great development with the chest lagging behind.

Lately, I have used another advanced technique called linear variable resistance training. Basically, either a heavy chain or elastic bands are attached to each end of the bar on a pressing movement. This makes the weights progressively heavier as you get closer to the top of the rep. This puts more resistance on the muscle, in turn recruiting more muscle fiber; which potentially means more growth.

No lagging behind today—or letting your chest hang low. Give these exercises a try and see the results for yourself!

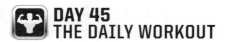

DAY 45
THE DAILY WORKOUT

THE MUSCLE BUILDER: LEGS
(Take 45 seconds - 1 minute rest between each set)
Lying leg curls – 5 sets of 10-12 reps
Stiff-legged deadlifts – 4 sets of 10-12 reps
Leg extensions – 5 sets of 10-12 reps (double drop set on last set)
45-degree Leg Press – 4 sets of 15 reps (double drop set on last set)
Hack Squat – 3 sets of 15 reps (triple drop set on last set)
Superset: Squats, walking lunges – 3 sets of 15-20 reps

CARDIO
20-30 minutes interval cardio on treadmill

HARDGAINER WORKOUT: REST

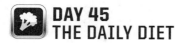

DAY 45
THE DAILY DIET

MEAL 1: Myofusion Shake: 2 scoops Myofusion, 1/2 cup egg whites, 2/3 cup instant oatmeal, 1 tablespoon natural peanut butter or almond butter, 1/2 cup apple juice, 1/2 cup water and ice.
MEAL 2: Myofusion Protein Pancakes: 1 scoop Myofusion, 1 cup egg hites, 1 cup oatmeal, 1/4 cup chopped walnuts, 1 sliced banana. Mix all together and cook on low heat on a non-stick pan using cooking spray. Optional: add sugar-free syrup.
MEAL 3: Same as Meal 1.
MEAL 4: 6 ounces canned tuna in spring water, 1 cup brown rice, 1 tablespoon olive oil or salad dressing with 1 cup veggies.
MEAL 5: Same as Meal 1.
MEAL 6: 8 ounces lean ground beef, 1 cup gluten-free pasta, 4-6 ounces low sodium natural tomato sauce with 1 tablespoon grated cheese *(optional)*.
MEAL 7 *(optional)*: Same as Meal 1.

DAY 45
THE DAILY TIP

There is nothing more impressive than a pair of striated, carved in stone, vascular pectoral muscles. By varying the angle of the incline bench in Incline Dumbbell Flyes, you can intentionally shift stress to specific areas of your upper-pectoral muscles. In Pec Deck Flyes, you can vary the stress of this movement—perform it with the seat set markedly higher or lower than normal.

You can also do the exercise with only one arm at a time—movements performed with one arm or leg at a time intensifies the stress of the exercise, since you no longer split your mental focus between two working limbs.

DAY 46 SHOW TIME!

There's nothing worse than preparing hard for something and then—at the moment your time to shine comes—falling flat on your face. Imagine studying all night for an exam and then falling asleep when the tests are handed out. Imagine learning everything about a company so you can do a great job interview, then realizing you had spinach stuck between your teeth when you met with the prospective boss. Imagine practicing shots from everywhere on the basketball court for hours a day, but then missing a game-winning free throw with seconds to go in the game.

Fifteen different times in my career I was named champion of a contest I was in. I didn't meet all my goals, but I came pretty darn close. I've always been a strong game day performer. I know how to close. So fast-forward from my last contest in 1996—12th place in the Florida Cup Pro and not the way I wanted to end my years of competing—to last July when it was time for the photo shoot I had just spent 51 days preparing for. I had worked my tail off getting ready and you better believe I was going to finish the job and be at my very best on photo shoot day.

My first photo shoot was scheduled on a Thursday at Mike Neveaux's studio. It was basically a private shoot with only a couple people there. For one week straight before the big day, I drank over a gallon of water each day to increase my ability to release more water. In other words, I needed to urinate more to dry out and look harder. I also restricted sodium for 2 days to release more water and the day of the shoot, I took in sodium and simple sugars by eating a cheese omelet with pancakes and syrup. It was the best breakfast I'd had in a long time, since all I'd had each morning for the previous 51 days were shakes.

I got to the studio parking lot in Gardena, California, and sat there for 15 minutes saying to myself, "The time is finally here." I was about to reveal the new trained and competition-level Rich Gaspari to the world, 15 years after my last photo shoot. Now I know many bodybuilders can say they look great, yet they don't deliver. I didn't want this to be me.

When I got to the dressing room, I put on shorts and still had no shirt on, but what I could see in the dressing room mirror was that I was both dry and ripped, and had veins everywhere like I always did in the old days. I hit some poses and saw I was getting even more pumped and full. I ended up shooting many different exercises as well as poses that day. It brought back all the memories of my past and the photo shoots I did back in the old days. It was like riding a bike. It all came back to me, and I was having a ball.

Now of course I was still in bodybuilder mode as well, so the whole time at the shoot I had to eat my meals to keep my body from going flat and stay full throughout the whole day. The photo shoot started at 10:00 a.m. and I shot photos and did interviews until 7:00 p.m. It was a long day to say the least, and I felt sore and tired from all the posing I did. I knew I also had another long photo shoot scheduled for the next day, so I made sure I ate well, staying basically on my diet and went to sleep early for my photo shoot at 9:00 a.m. in Venice Gold's Gym. The Mecca!

Now this was very exciting because this time the photo shoot was to be in the gym I trained in when I competed in the Mr. Olympia, and many people would be there watching me to see how I looked after many years away from the stage. We took many shots similar to my old pictures to compare my condition then and now.

It was a really exciting moment in my life to be photographed in the gym I had trained in during my twenties. Now in my late forties I was back at the same place to be photographed again. Several people in the gym I knew from twenty years ago were shaking their heads in disbelief that I was back in competition shape. It was a great feeling for so many people to come up to me and say I looked fantastic and that it was as though time had stood still.

You've been on this journey now for close to seven weeks. It's time for you to show yourself to the world. It might not be a photo shoot or a contest. It might be a pool party or outdoor event. If you haven't planned it—do so now. I want you to go show people what you've accomplished. No false modesty. If you were finishing up college you would go to your graduation ceremony, wouldn't you? You didn't start this to get halfway there. Now is the time to dig in and finish the job. It's show time!

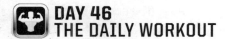
DAY 46
THE DAILY WORKOUT

THE MUSCLE BUILDER: SHOULDERS & ABS
(Take 45 seconds - 1 minute rest between each set)

Seated barbell front press – 4 sets of 8-12 reps

Giantset: Seated side laterals, Arnold Press, Standing dumbbell upright rows – 4 sets of 10-12 reps

Incline one arm side laterals – 3 sets of 12-15

Machine rear laterals – 4 sets of 12-15

Barbell shrugs from behind – 4 sets of 12-15

Twisting crunches – 4 sets of 30 reps

Leg raises – 4 sets of 25 reps

CARDIO
20-30 minutes interval cardio on treadmill

HARDGAINER WORKOUT: CHEST/BACK/BICEPS/TRICEPS/ABS
Modified Compound Superset #1

Flat Dumbbell Bench Press: 3 sets of 8, 6, 4 reps (90 second rest)

Close Grip Neutral Grip Pull-Ups: 3 sets of 8, 6, 4 reps (Strap weight on if you can – 2 mins rest)

Note: If you cannot perform the Close Grip Pull-Up, either have someone spot you by using your legs off their hands for leverage or have them spot-push you up by the waist.

Modified Compound Superset #2

Incline Barbell Bench Press: 3 sets of 8, 6, 4 reps (90 second rest)

Bent Over Underhand Barbell Row: 3 sets of 8, 6, 4 reps (2 min rest)

Giant Modified Compound Super Set #3 – *Take prescribed rest between exercise*

Chest Dips: 3 sets of 8, 6, 4 reps (60 second rest)

Preacher Curls: 3 sets of 8, 6, 4 reps (45 second rest)

Close Grip Bench Press: 3 sets of 8, 6, 4 reps (2 min rest)

Giant Modified Compound Super Set #4

E-Z Preacher Curls: 3 sets of 8, 6, 4 reps (60 second rest)

Lying Triceps Extensions: 3 sets of 8, 6, 4 reps (45 second rest)
Swiss Ball (aka "Inflated Fitness Ball") Crunches: 3 sets of 20, 15, 10
   reps (Hold a weight plate or dumbbell overhead if you can)
   (2 min rest)

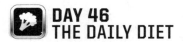

DAY 46
THE DAILY DIET

MEAL 1: Myofusion Shake: 2 scoops Myofusion, 1/2 cup egg whites, 2/3
   cup instant oatmeal, 1 tablespoon natural peanut butter or
   almond butter, 1/2 cup apple juice, 1/2 cup water and ice.
MEAL 2: Myofusion Protein Pancakes: 1 scoop Myofusion, 1 cup egg
   whites, 1 cup oatmeal, 1/4 cup chopped walnuts, 1 sliced
   banana. Mix all together and cook on low heat on a non-stick
   pan using cooking spray. Optional: add sugar-free syrup.
MEAL 3: Same as Meal 1.
MEAL 4: 8 ounces lean buffalo patty *(or 93% lean ground beef)* with
   salsa or mustard, 1 cup
   brown rice, 6 ounces green salad with vinegar.
MEAL 5: 10 raw almonds.
MEAL 6: Egg omelet: 1 cup egg whites mixed with 1 cup chopped
   peppers, onions, and tomatoes. 6 ounces green salad with
   vinegar, and 1 slice watermelon on the side.
MEAL 7 *(optional)***:** Same as Meal 1.

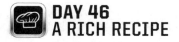

DAY 46
A RICH RECIPE

QUICK-GATOR SMOOTHIE

2 cups ice

*1 serving orange Gaspari Nutrition Glycofuse
   (or substitute your favorite flavor)*

*2 – 3 scoops Gaspari Nutrition Delicious Orange Cream
   or Vanilla Isofusion*

2 cups of water

Combine all ingredients in a blender and blend until smooth.
Pour into glasses and serve immediately. Makes 2 servings.

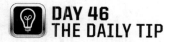 **DAY 46
THE DAILY TIP**

*Learn all you can about macronutrients: proteins, carbohydrates, and
fats. For example, when most people who are trying to get fit hear the
word "fats" they freak out and run the other direction. Well you can't
burn fat if you don't ingest fat. The key is the right kind of fat. This book
is just an appetizer on good nutrition.*

DAY 47 A FOUR-LETTER WORD

For millions of Americans, the word "diet" is a four-letter word that brings up all sorts of negative connotations: Self-denial. Deprivation. Hunger. Cravings. Unrealized expectations. Uncontrolled binges. Failure. Yet our overweight nation spends billions of dollars every year trying to find the magic pill or the latest diet fad that promises to melt away the pounds. I've said it before—and it certainly applies here—nothing worth having is easy. Cutting back on your caloric intake in order to achieve your ultimate body is not going to be a walk in the park. Giving up the unhealthy foods you crave is not going to be easy.

But here's the good news: if you stick to the plan you certainly aren't going to go hungry. Seven meals a day means you eat every two and a half hours during your waking hours. Your problem isn't going to be hunger. The challenge is going to be making good food choices and finding the time to prepare and eat all of those meals on schedule.

It's a lot of work to prepare seven meals a day and then take time to eat them. When I'm really busy, one of my meals during the day will be a protein shake. They are fast and easy and keep me on my plan. And although I put in a lot of hours at work, the good thing for me is I'm the boss. If I want to microwave one of the meals I prepared the night before and eat it in the middle of a meeting I can do it without hurting my career. I may be driving everyone crazy, but everyone that works with me knows I'm a little crazy when it comes to my workout regimes anyway.

One of the biggest challenges I used to face as a competitor and then as CEO of a company was eating on the road. Whenever I travel, my first stop was always the grocery store. Why? I made my own meals in my hotel room. When I booked my travel itinerary, I wasn't worried about how luxurious my room would be—I just wanted to make sure there was a refrigerator and microwave in the room.

Fortunately, things are much better now. Restaurants have begun offering leaner, healthier options. If you are a road warrior like me, you can stay on the diet and still eat at restaurants—as long as you make the right choices. Eating grilled chicken with a green salad is great. Make sure you choose a vinaigrette dressing or just plain oil and vinegar on the side. If you have a power meal at a steak house, a lean filet mignon, grilled fish (especially salmon with all those Omega-3 oils), plain baked potatoes, steamed vegetables—there are plenty of good choices. It's even possible to eat out at fast food places now. That doesn't mean you can order anything on the board. But many offer grilled chicken and salads, as well as other lean choices.

Obviously, you need to be staying away from white flour and sugar products. These foods are highly processed and offer little nutritional value, not to mention they tend to be high in starches and calories—and highly addictive. Instead, look for products made with whole grains, such as replacing white sandwich bread with whole grain bread. Whole grains have the added benefit of providing you with plenty of fiber. Perhaps you have a sweet tooth and love desert. Look online for alternative recipes for cakes, pies, muffins, puddings, and other things you love using low-calorie, natural sweeteners like stevia.

Another step that I took for my transformation was eating a gluten-free diet. Gluten is a protein which is present in grains of wheat, rye, barley, and oats. For some, such as those with Celiac disease, avoiding gluten is a life and death necessity. For others with a gluten sensitivity, avoiding gluten can help reduce digestive distress, respiratory allergies, and chronic pain, as well a wide range of other problems.

But as long as you don't indulge in gluten-free versions of those same processed, high-sugar, high-carbohydrate foods (breads, muffins, brownies, etc.), and you eat plenty of complex carbohydrate grains, such as brown rice and quinoa, a gluten-free diet can be particularly helpful in building lean muscle mass and losing weight.

Achieving your ultimate body isn't just about working out smarter and harder than you ever have before. It's also about changing how you eat. Not a month-long diet, not a 51-day diet, but a new lifestyle. Get rid of any negative thoughts you have about the word "diet" right now. Don't just go through the motions on the diet portion of this program. Get into it. Embrace it. Who knows, you might just end up loving not only your new body—but the new way of feeding it!

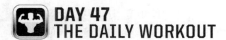 **DAY 47**
THE DAILY WORKOUT

THE MUSCLE BUILDER: BICEPS & TRICEPS
[Take 45 seconds - 1 minute rest between each set]

Superset: Incline dumbbell curls, Rope pushdowns – 4 sets of 10 reps

Superset: Standing barbell curls, Seated 2-arm overhead tricep extension with Dumbbell – 4 sets of 10 reps

Superset: Seated preacher curls with EZ curl bar, Lying pullover press – 4 sets of 10 reps

Superset: Dumbbell concentration curls, cable kickbacks – 4 sets of 10 reps

CARDIO
20-30 minutes interval cardio on treadmill

HARDGAINER WORKOUT: THIGHS/HAMSTRINGS/DELTS/CALVES
Modified Compound Superset #1

Medium Stance Squats: 3 sets of 8, 6, 4 reps [90 second rest]

Lying Leg Curls: 3 sets of 8, 6, 4 reps [90 second rest]

Note: If you suffer from lower back problems you may substitute the squat for the leg press. Since you are performing the leg press as your second exercise, then just use a close stance on this one and a medium stance on the second one.

Modified Compound Superset #2

Leg Press: 3 sets of 8, 6, 4 reps [90 second rest]

Barbell Romanian Deadlifts: 3 sets of 8, 6, 4 reps [2 min rest]

Modified Compound Superset #3

Seated Barbell Front Shoulder: 3 sets of 8, 6, 4 reps [60 second rest]

Standing Calf Raise (Gastrocs): 3 sets of 10, 8, 6 reps [2 min rest]

Modified Compound Superset #4

Dumbbell Lateral Raises: 3 sets of 8, 6, 4 reps [60 second rest]

Lying Leg Raises with a pop at the top of each rep: 3 sets of 10, 8, 6 reps [60 second rest]

Descending Set #5 – *Drop the weight as you move from set-to-set*
Seated Calf Raises (Soleus) - 3 Descending Sets – Decrease weight as
you descend, if necessary:
- 1st set of 12-15 reps (15 sec rest)
- 2nd set of 12-15 reps (15 sec rest)
- 3rd set of 12-15 reps (1 min rest & repeat 2 more times)

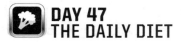

DAY 47
THE DAILY DIET

MEAL 1: Myofusion Shake: 2 scoops Myofusion, 1/2 cup egg whites,
2/3 cup instant oatmeal, 1 tablespoon natural peanut butter
or almond butter, 1/2 cup apple juice, 1/2 cup water and ice.

MEAL 2: Myofusion Protein Pancakes: 1 scoop Myofusion, 1 cup egg
whites, 1 cup oatmeal, 1/4 cup chopped walnuts, 1 sliced
banana. Mix all together and cook on low heat on a non-stick
pan using cooking spray. Optional: add sugar-free syrup.

MEAL 3: Same as Meal 1.

MEAL 4: 8 ounces grilled chicken breast, 1 cup brown rice, 1 cup
steamed broccoli.

MEAL 5: Same as Meal 1.

MEAL 6: 8 ounces mahi mahi or other white fish, 1 small potato,
3 ounces steamed string beans, 4 ounces green salad
with vinegar.

MEAL 7 *(optional)***:** Same as Meal 1.

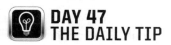

DAY 47
THE DAILY TIP

*The hardest time of year to stay in shape is the holidays. How do you
handle this season of feasting and festivities? It's all about good habits.
Consider piling up the lean turkey, and go easy on the candied yams, pies,
cakes, and other refined carbs and high-fat foods. If you have been able
to get into the healthy nutritional habits of eating low fat, high quality
proteins, unrefined complex carbs, whole fruits, and healthy fats, give
yourself permission to splurge here and there. Just don't go overboard!*

DAY 48 RELATIONSHIP EQUITY

After growing up in humble circumstances, fighting my way to the top of a high visibility sport and gaining some level of celebrity status, crashing and burning financially, and then making a slow and steady climb to the top of the sports nutrition industry, I have some simple advice for you: be careful how you treat people when you are on your way up. Because you might see them again on your way down!

Do I like my office better now than when I worked out of my mom's basement? Do I appreciate having a state-of-the-art warehouse more than having to store my inventory in her garage? No doubt. But you know what? I believe I was the same person then that I am now. I am just as proud of the Rich who was struggling to get something off the ground as I am of the leader I've become. And I believe I have treated people with interest, respect, and consideration whether I was up or down. If you think I'm not remembering things correctly, I would love for you to write or email me. If I owe anyone an apology, I am man enough to do it.

I can't say I was treated the same way by everyone I worked with and even considered a friend. There weren't many issues for me before I had my professional break-through. After all, I was an eager young pup with bound-less energy and enthusiasm and people could see I was going to accomplish things. Oh, there were a few people who tried to put me in my place both one-on-one and in the media. But that's to be expected in any competitive endeavor. I never took anything too personally.

But when my career was torpedoed by injury and then a few bad business decisions, some folks showed their true colors. The claws came out. I don't know what hurt more—being ignored or being ripped or having people feel sorry for me. Am I writing this because I'm bitter? Am I going to mention names and get some revenge? Nope. Even if I tried, I'm not sure I could hold a grudge. I still see some of the people who were hardest on me at contests and exhibits and we act like we've never been anything but good friends. I'm 100% fine with that. It's all water under the bridge.

The reason this topic is so important to me is that as much as I love competition and winning, I still believe one of the most important choices we make is how we treat others. What good does it do you to build a huge muscular, impressive body if you are small and underdeveloped on the inside? I've always felt that success begins on the inside and reaching our true potential gets blocked when we are small-spirited.

The truth is, no one admires a big bully, but everyone is impressed with someone who is big, strong, and powerful—*and* kind. This program carries far outside of the gym and spills over into all of your life. It is about hard work, determination, learning, and making good choices.

Treat people right. You may not get the response or same treatment immediately. But over time, you will build relationship equity. Nothing else will promote your personal success better than that.

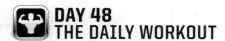

DAY 48
THE DAILY WORKOUT

THE MUSCLE BUILDER: REST

HARDGAINER WORKOUT: REST

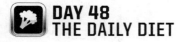

DAY 48
THE DAILY DIET

MEAL 1: Myofusion Shake: 2 scoops Myofusion, 1/2 cup egg whites, 2/3 cup instant oatmeal, 1 tablespoon natural peanut butter or almond butter, 1/2 cup apple juice, 1/2 cup water and ice.

MEAL 2: Myofusion Protein Pancakes: 1 scoop Myofusion, 1 cup egg whites, 1 cup oatmeal, 1/4 cup chopped walnuts, 1 sliced banana. Mix all together and cook on low heat on a non-stick pan using cooking spray. Optional: add sugar-free syrup.

MEAL 3: Same as Meal 1.

MEAL 4: Egg omelet: 1 cup egg whites mixed with 1 cup chopped peppers, onions, and tomatoes. 6 ounces green salad with vinegar, and 1 apple on the side.

MEAL 5: Same as Meal 1.

MEAL 6: 8 ounces of lean steak, 1 sweet potato, 1 cup raw kale salad with 1 teaspoon olive oil and lemon juice.

MEAL 7 *(optional)*: Same as Meal 1.

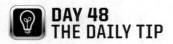

DAY 48
THE DAILY TIP

Excuse: *I don't feel motivated enough.* **Answer:** *Sure, training can be boring at times, but exercise is not always about doing 3 sets of 8-12 reps. If you're sick and tired of traditional weight training, there are other options to become bigger, leaner, and stronger. Switch things up and watch what happens!*

DAY 49 ONE STEP AT A TIME

Instant gratification is great if you can get it. But for most of us success comes in baby steps. I think this is hard for a lot of us to accept because we live in such a prosperous country that is filled with conveniences. Now there have been a few years of recession and many young people have learned you can't just graduate from college and get a starting salary making $80,000 or $100,000 or more. Millions of people have overspent and over-borrowed getting things they should have saved up for first. And they've felt the pinch. When I was in high school and then went off to Rutgers University, I didn't have any expectation of driving a nice set of wheels. I drove a beater and didn't think anything about it. I knew that success was achieved one step at a time.

If you want to make it in bodybuilding, there's a pretty set pattern everyone follows. You compete as an amateur in a local show, then move up to a regional or state show, and maybe after a few years, you can qualify for a national show. I was one of the fortunate ones that earned my pro card the first time I competed nationally as an amateur. That was an incredible experience, but I didn't let it go to my head. I was expecting it would take another year or two.

It was the same in my life as an entrepreneur. First, I sold other people's supplements to clients I trained. Then I was able to get a supplier to give me a good deal on a line of private label supplements. That was when I was able to add a few local stores. My stuff sat on the shelf in some stores but I had a few owners and managers that got behind what I was trying to do and gave me a boost by promoting it word-of-mouth with their customers. It took another year to move beyond private label supplements and actually find a compounder to make my own formulas. Then it took a couple more years until I was able to hook up with a national distributor. When I look back, I can't believe that I am coming up on 15 years and my products are now being sold in more than 70 countries.

I don't say this to brag or try to make anyone jealous. I am both proud and humbled. I know that not all ideas pan out. As an entrepreneur, I've had months where I had no clue how I was going to make ends meet. But I learned a couple of lessons along the way. First, you can't quit pursuing your dreams. The moment you quit you have guaranteed failure. You will wonder the rest of your life if you should have fought on a little bit longer. Secondly, as I've already mentioned, success is usually incremental. Yes, sometimes someone writes their first book and it becomes a huge bestseller. The same thing happens in music. But sometimes what we think is an immediate success story really has a long trail of blood, sweat, and tears that led up to it. All we see is that breakthrough moment. We don't realize that most success stories include paying one's dues.

The Chinese philosopher Lao-tzu maybe said it best: "A journey of a thousand miles begins with a single step." On Day 1 of this journey, I challenged you to simply start where you were. That principle is just as true today as it was then. Today the slate is wiped clean and the only question is are you going to quit or take another step? Big doesn't happen overnight. At least not the substantial "big" that is based on real muscle gain. If someone promises you their product will shed 20 pounds and give you a lean hard body with no work and in very little time—run! It's a step-by-step journey.

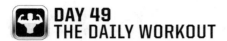

DAY 49
THE DAILY WORKOUT

THE MUSCLE BUILDER: REST

HARDGAINER WORKOUT: REST

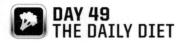

DAY 49
THE DAILY DIET

MEAL 1: Myofusion Shake: 2 scoops Myofusion, 1/2 cup egg whites, 2/3 cup instant oatmeal, 1 tablespoon natural peanut butter or almond butter, 1/2 cup apple juice, 1/2 cup water and ice.

MEAL 2: Myofusion Protein Pancakes: 1 scoop Myofusion, 1 cup egg Whites, 1 cup oatmeal, 1/4 cup chopped walnuts, 1 sliced banana. Mix all together and cook on low heat on a non-stick pan using cooking spray. Optional: add sugar-free syrup.

MEAL 3: Same as Meal 1.

MEAL 4: 8 ounces grilled tuna, 1 cup brown rice, 1 teaspoon of olive oil, 1 cup steamed green beans.

MEAL 5: 10 raw almonds.

MEAL 6: 8 ounces lean ground beef, 1 cup gluten-free pasta, 4-6 ounces low sodium natural tomato sauce with 1 tablespoon grated cheese *[optional]*.

MEAL 7 *[optional]*: Same as Meal 1.

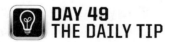

DAY 49
THE DAILY TIP

Arnold presses, made famous by Mr. Schwarzenegger himself, shock the delts. To do this exercise, you either sit or stand, holding dumbbells at your shoulders with your palms turned in toward your body—as in the top of a dumbbell curl. As you press the dumbbells overhead, twist your hands so your palms face each other about halfway up and face forward at the top. It's important to avoid fully locking out at the top so you get constant tension on your delts.

DAY 50 YOUR NUMBER ONE PRIORITY

In the June 2011 issue of *Muscle Sport magazine*, my good friend and a great writer, Joe Pietaro, asked me point blank what a lot of people were wondering at the time: "Are you making a comeback to competitive bodybuilding?" We had seen each other at my induction into Muscle Beach Hall of Fame and it was no secret I was training to appear on the cover of *Iron Man*. No matter what I said to the contrary, rumors were swirling that I was going to compete again.

I got my butt kicked by Albert Beckles in 1985 when I was 20 years old. He was 50. So I knew firsthand it is possible to compete at age 48. But what Joe and others thought was that more than likely I would join the Masters Division to compete against some great friends and rivals from my glory years. When I saw the lineup of legends that were committed to compete in December, 2011, at the IFBB Pro World Master Championship in Miami Beach, I did a double-take. What a blast it would be to get up there and fight it out and pose alongside greats like Ronnie Coleman, Samir Bannout, Dexter Jackson, Stan Frydrych, Andreas Cahling, Chris Cormier, Pavol Jablonicky, Roland Czuirlock, Toney Freeman, Troy Alves, Dennis James, Darrem Charles, Gary Strydom, Lee Apperson, Bill Wilmore, Lawrence Hunt, and others. And my good friend Shawn Ray was hosting the event too.

Who knows, if Lee Haney was on the platform I might have changed my mind just to try one more time to beat him. We may be like brothers, but we all know brothers can mix it up at times. The Pro Masters circuit hasn't had quite as much traction with fans the past few years, but it's still a strong and popular enterprise with a lot of potential to grow. And this past year had the most impressive lineup yet. I was honored and humbled when Joe told me he thought I could bring some extra appeal to the Masters.

So I'm going to put my absolute ironclad answer out there to settle the question hopefully once and for all. I guess you can never say never—okay, I'm really just kidding when I say that—but I feel I had my day in the spotlight as a competitor. I may miss it like crazy sometimes, but that era for Rich Gaspari is over. Maybe I would team up with some friends to "guest pose" at some competitions, but my days as a bodybuilding competitor are finished. And the reason is simple. It's not that I'm not driven to achieve my ultimate body. I think I've proved that this past year. I got in better form than anyone thought possible—and I've kept it. I think I'm smart enough and strategic enough to avoid the injuries that plagued me the last few years of my pro career, so fear of injury isn't it. I haven't lost one scintilla of passion for the sport I love. So it's not that I've lost interest.

To put it simply—I love what I'm doing. I'm passionate about growing my company. I compete my butt off every day. Keeping a highly talented staff pulling in the same direction is probably the biggest challenge I've ever encountered in my adult working life. It's not because my people are unmotivated and lack ideas. It's the opposite. I've got a group of war horses that are ready to go to battle every day. They have more great ideas than I can keep up with. I feel like the cowboy in the commercial a couple of years ago who had to herd rabbits. My team is smart, fast, and agile. So I have to make sure we have the production capacity and cash flow to do all we want to do. It's a whole different world than trying to get my calves to respond to training!

I still think I'm a comeback kid, it just won't be as a bodybuilding competitor. I've got enough experience and maturity to know that life requires the tough task of prioritization. I'll always believe you and I can accomplish the impossible—but I've been around the block a few times and know there are only 24 hours in a day. I'm thankful for all the opportunities I have, but I know not all opportunities are created equal and

I have to make tough decisions. Personal bodybuilding is still a huge priority for me. This may surprise people, but I believe taking my company to the next level is even bigger. I think I can do even more for the sport by keeping Gaspari Nutrition a healthy dynamic force for good.

I'm a driven goal-oriented person. I've been asked a number of times if I'd sell my company so I could sit back and enjoy the financial rewards of that move. My response is always the same. If I wasn't driving and striving, I'd be bored out of my mind. My advice to you is to keep your eyes open for the opportunities that are all around you. Then force yourself to determine which of those opportunities is best for you.

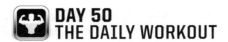 **DAY 50**
THE DAILY WORKOUT

THE MUSCLE BUILDER: CHEST & ABS
(Take 45 seconds - 1 minute rest between each set)
Incline dumbbell press – 4 sets of 8-10 reps
Incline dumbbell flies – 4 sets of 8-10 reps
Decline cable flies – 4 sets of 8-10 reps
Superset: Dumbbell flat bench, Pec Dec – 4 sets of 8-10 reps
Crunches – 4 sets of 25-30 reps
Leg raises – 4 sets of 25-30 reps

CARDIO
20-30 minutes interval cardio on treadmill

HARDGAINER WORKOUT: CHEST/BACK/BICEPS/TRICEPS/CORE
Modified Compound Superset #1 – *Take 45 seconds rest before moving on to the 2nd exercise*
Incline Dumbbell Press: 3 sets of 4-6 reps (45 Sec Rest)
Barbell Bent Over Row: 3 sets of 4-6 reps (1 min rest)
Modified Compound Superset #2 – *Take 45 seconds rest before moving on to the 2nd exercise*
Flat Dumbbell Bench Press: 3 sets of 6-8 reps (45 Sec Rest)
Chin-Ups: 3 sets of 6-8 reps (Strap on weight if you can)(1 min rest)
   Note: If you cannot perform the Chin-up, either have someone spot you by using your legs off their hands for leverage or have them spot-push you up by the waist.
Superset #3 – *No rest between exercises*
Barbell Curls: 3 sets of 8-10 reps (No Rest)
Close Grip Dumbbell Bench Press (Triceps): 3 sets of 8-10 reps (1 min rest)
Superset #4 – *No rest between exercises*
Dumbbell Hammer Curls: 3 sets of 10-12 reps (No Rest)
Triceps Pushdowns: 3 sets of 10-12 reps (1 min rest)
Superset #4 – *No rest between exercises*

Plank: 2 sets of 1 Minute Static Contraction (No Rest)
Bicycle Maneuver: 2 sets of 30 reps (1 min rest)

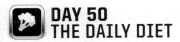

DAY 50
THE DAILY DIET

MEAL 1: Myofusion Shake: 2 scoops Myofusion, 1/2 cup egg whites, 2/3 cup instant oatmeal, 1 tablespoon natural peanut butter or almond butter, 1/2 cup apple juice, 1/2 cup water and ice.

MEAL 2: Myofusion Protein Pancakes: 1 scoop Myofusion, 1 cup egg whites, 1 cup oatmeal, 1/4 cup chopped walnuts, 1 sliced banana. Mix all together and cook on low heat on a non-stick pan using cooking spray. Optional: add sugar-free syrup.

MEAL 3: 10 raw almonds.

MEAL 4: 8 ounces grilled chicken, 1 cup brown rice, 1 tablespoon olive oil or salad dressing with 1 cup veggies.

MEAL 5: Same as Meal 1.

MEAL 6: 8 ounces lean buffalo patty (or 93% lean ground beef) with salsa or mustard, 1 small potato, 1 cup raw kale salad with 1 teaspoon olive oil and lemon juice.

MEAL 7 (optional): Same as Meal 1.

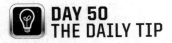

DAY 50
THE DAILY TIP

The abdominal muscles and the rest of the core musculature is considered the epicenter of the human body—but the core is made up of more than just the abs and includes the back and hips. More than just about good looks—a solid core translates into almost all of your daily physical activities. Strengthening your entire core will help you achieve optimal performance while reducing the risk of physical injuries during physical activities.

DAY 51 THE FUTURE IS NOW

There's a saying in college football that I like: "You can't win a national championship during spring training, but you can sure lose one." I also like to repeat the old quote that championships are won when no one is watching.

We all love when it's game day and the lights come up. I always loved show time. But the reason I didn't have big problems with nerves is that I knew I had done my very best to prepare. Someone might be better than me, but not because I hadn't done everything in my power to get ready. You see, show time doesn't really begin on the day a competition is scheduled on the calendar. It is a year round endeavor.

The three months prior to any competition, my intensity was incredible. I would fly back to California. The gyms were more intense and it was a good time to work with the industry media on photo shoots and just overall networking. But those three months weren't spent soaking up the sunshine and enjoying the beach. It was all work. Whenever the question of who had the best work ethic comes up in bodybuilding circles, even in current articles, my name is on the short list and usually near the top.

Everyday you are faced with choices that determine your future—so why not make a choice that makes your future a better place? That's the heart of the matter. That's what preparation is: making choices today that will enhance your future when it's game on. You don't work out today because of what you're gong to achieve before you go to bed. You work out today because of what it will give you when you are performing in the spotlight.

The reason some people get in such a hurry and do crazy things to get in shape is that they don't understand the principle of time. The future isn't 51 days from now. It is *today*. I don't know how many people I've seen try to gain a level of mass in a couple months that it takes a year to build. They'll get on a crazy supplement and actually get a lot bigger. They really believe they've found a secret to cheat time. But it's all fat and excess water weight. When they have to drop pounds for a competition to get shredded they discover there's not enough real muscle underneath to get defined. They're still trying to carve a sculpture out of a twig. Mass is something you build one day at a time. So if you want to gain 20 pounds of muscle for next fall, you had better start today.

When someone asked stock market guru Warren Buffett how long he likes to hold onto a stock, his answer was, "forever." He made billions because he both understood the principle of time and invested in people who had the same understanding. He didn't become a billionaire by being a day trader. He built his fortune by applying sound principles and letting time do its work. From 2000-2010 his stock yielded a 76% return versus the S&P average of -11%. One share of Berkshire Hathaway stock costs almost $120,000 —highest on the NYSE. You don't achieve numbers like Buffett has without working harder and smarter every single day. He didn't believe in overnight success with investing and I sure don't with bodybuilding.

When it comes to the future, some people believe in luck and others believe in fate. My belief is real simple. I believe in preparation. What you are tomorrow won't be by accident. You will be the sum total of the decisions and actions you make each day.

Based on your workouts this past week and assuming you continue a the same pace, what are you gong to look like one week from now? One month? One year? Are you going to like the way you look or are you gong to wish you had pushed harder? If you don't like the answer, just realize the choice to change the future in your hands. The future begins right now.

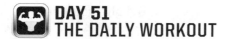 **DAY 51**
THE DAILY WORKOUT

THE MUSCLE BUILDER: BACK & CALVES
(Take 45 seconds - 1 minute rest between each set)
Deadlifts – 4 sets of 8-10 reps
Wide grip chins – 4 sets of 8-10 reps
Superset: Close grip pulldowns, Wide grip cable pullovers – 4 sets of 8-10 reps
Superset: Cable low rows, T-bar rows – 4 sets of 8-10 reps
Superset: Two arm dumbbell rows, machine rows – 4 sets of 8-10 reps
Standing Calf raises – 5 sets of 15 reps
Seated calf raises – 5 sets of 15 reps

CARDIO
20-30 minutes interval cardio on treadmill

HARDGAINER WORKOUT:
THIGHS/HAMSTRINGS/DELTS/CALVES/LOWER ABS
Superset #1
Wide Stance Squats: 3 sets of 4-6 reps (45 Seconds Rest)
Stiff Legged Barbell Deadlifts: 3 sets of 4-6 reps (1 min rest)
> *Note: Utilize the "Full Body Tension Technique": This is when you stay in proper anatomical form and maintain that posture by keeping all of your major muscles contracted before & throughout the movements. This will keep you safe, while allowing you to use maximum intensity.*

Giant Set #2 – *3 exercises performed back-to-back without rest*
Leg Press: 3 sets of 6-8 reps (No Rest)
Leg Extensions: 3 sets of 10-12 reps (No Rest)
Lying Leg Curls: 3 sets of 10-12 reps (1 min rest)
Giant Set #3
Upright Barbell Row: 3 sets of 8-10 reps (No Rest)
Lateral Raises: 3 sets of 8-10 reps (No Rest)

Descending Set #4 – *Drop the weight as you move from set-to-set*
Standing Calf Raises (Gastrocs) - 3 Descending Sets – Decrease
weight as you descend, if necessary:
- 1st set of 12-15 reps (15 sec rest)
- 2nd set of 12-15 reps (15 sec rest)
- 3rd set of 12-15 reps (1 min rest & repeat 2 more times)

Superset #5
Bent Over Lateral Dumbbell Raises: 3 sets of 10-12 reps (No Rest)
Seated Calf Raises (Soleus): 3 sets of 10-12 reps (1 min rest)
Hanging Leg Raises: 3 sets of 15-20 reps (1 min rest)

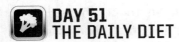 ## DAY 51
THE DAILY DIET

MEAL 1: Myofusion Shake: 2 scoops Myofusion, 1/2 cup egg whites,
2/3 cup instant oatmeal, 1 tablespoon natural peanut butter
or almond butter, 1/2 cup apple juice, 1/2 cup water and ice.

MEAL 2: Myofusion Protein Pancakes: 1 scoop Myofusion, 1 cup egg
whites, 1 cup oatmeal, 1/4 cup chopped walnuts, 1 sliced
banana. Mix all together and cook on low heat on a non-stick
pan using cooking spray. Optional: add sugar-free syrup.

MEAL 3: Same as Meal 1.

MEAL 4: 8 ounce grilled chicken, 1 cup brown rice, 1 tablespoon olive oil
or salad dressing with 1 cup veggies.

MEAL 5: 10 raw almonds.

MEAL 6: 8 ounce of lean steak, 1 sweet potato, 1 cup raw kale salad
with 1 teaspoon olive oil and lemon juice.

MEAL 7 [optional]**:** Same as Meal 1.

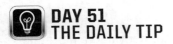 ## DAY 51
THE DAILY TIP

Always look forward into the future—your past is behind you for a reason.

APPENDIX FOOD AND SUPPLEMENTS

While contouring the outside of the body, it is also imperative to control what goes inside your body. Foods can be divided into three primary macronutrient groups defined as the classes of chemical compounds humans consume in the largest quantities and which provide bulk energy. These are proteins, fats, and carbohydrates. Fiber, a non-digestible carbohydrate deserves its own mention.

When food doesn't provide all the nutrients needed for health, we must carefully add well-chosen vitamins and minerals. Not just any bottle will do. Reading labels and doing your research will add those helpful nutrients to your diet.

Supplementing amino acids will add greatly to your workout and your efforts at building a healthier you. Hunted down for you is a list of healthy amino acids that will give you a stronger and more productive workout.

MACRONUTRIENTS

PROTEINS
Every cell, tissue, and organ in our body contain protein. These proteins are continually being broken down and needing to be replaced. Proteins are actually made up of amino acids, which are called the building blocks of our body tissue.

There are 20 different types of amino acids and they are divided into three groups: *essential amino acids, non-essential amino acids,* and *conditional amino acids.*

Essential amino acids cannot be made by the body. Therefore, it is essential to have them in our diet. Non-essential amino acids are made by the body from essential amino acids. And conditional amino acids are only needed during time of illness or stress.

Protein sources are grouped according to how many essential amino acids they contain. Complete proteins contain all of the essential amino acids. Animal-based foods like meat, chicken, fish, eggs, milk and cheese would be considered complete proteins. Incomplete protein sources lack one or more of the essential amino acids. Complementary protein sources contain two or more proteins that together contain all the necessary essential amino acids.

CARBOHYDRATES

The main role of carbohydrates is to provide energy to the cells of the body. There are three forms of carbohydrates: simple carbs (sugars), complex carbs (starches), and fiber. The Recommended Daily Allowance (RDA) is for 130 grams per day; however, most Americans ingest much more than this. The average intake is 220 to 330 grams per day (gpd) for men, and 180 to 230 for women. The excess carbohydrates are converted into glycogen and stored in the liver, or into glucose and stored in the blood. Excess carbs over the storage amount will be converted directly into fat.

Simple carbs—referred to as sugary foods—are found in fruits, milk and milk products, and vegetables. They are also found in refined and processed foods such as candy, soda, corn syrup, and table sugar. Refined sugars provide calories, but lack vitamins, minerals, and fiber. Such simple sugars are often called "empty calories" and can lead to weight gain.

Complex carbs—often referred to as "starchy" foods—include legumes, starchy vegetables and whole-grain breads and cereals. Fibrous carbs come from vegetables as well as fruits that contain a large amount of fiber.

Refined foods such as white flour, sugar, and white rice, have had important nutrients and fiber removed, so it is important to get your carbs as well as other foods in their natural form. Whole foods come in their natural whole state. They are a food that has not been refined, processed, or adulterated. Man-made refined foods are void of enzymes, trace elements *and* the naturally occurring vitamins *and* minerals in whole foods. Think whole grains instead of refined, a piece of fruit instead of juice, veggies with the peel, and others.

The Glycemic Index is a helpful tool that shows the blood glucose response to foods showing which foods raise the blood sugar level more quickly. Processed carbs, refined foods, and added sugars are more likely to raise your sugar level quickly. Whole unprocessed foods, that are digested more slowly, enter your bloodstream more slowly as well. Eating fat or protein with the carbohydrates will also slow digestion and decrease the GI content of the food.

FAT

Fat is a source of fuel energy and helps the body absorb fat-soluble vitamins. Fats are made up of four groups: mono-unsaturated fat, poly-unsaturated fat, saturated fat, and trans fat.

Mono-unsaturated fats have one double-carbon bond, as opposed to poly-unsaturated fats, which have multiple double bonds. These fats can reduce "bad" cholesterol in your blood. Monounsaturated fat is helpful for weight loss because it promotes the feeling of satiety, or fullness, making it easier to adhere to your diet plan. It can also reduce the risk of many types of cancers. Good dietary sources of mono-unsaturated fats include olive oil, canola oil, rapeseed oil, sesame oil, avocados, olives, and most nuts.

Poly-unsaturated fats have multiple double bonds. Double bonds are good because they eliminate hydrogen atoms. Both mono-unsaturated and poly-unsaturated oils are believed to lower cholesterol. Unsaturated fats remain liquid, even at low temperatures. Good sources include corn oil, soybean oil, safflower oil, tofu and soymilk, fatty fish like salmon, tuna, and mackerel, and seeds like sunflower and pumpkin.

Saturated fats include high fat meats like beef, pork, and chicken, as well as lard, whole fat milk products like milk, cream, butter, and cheese, and palm and coconut oil. Not all saturated fats are created equal. Saturated fats contain fatty acids such as lauric acid, myristic acid, and caprylic acid, which are antifungal, antimicrobial, and antiviral. All of these contribute towards a stronger immune system. More than half of the brain consists of saturated fat and cholesterol. Saturated fats are more heat stable than poly-unsaturated oils, which are likely to become rancid and oxidized and turn into cell-damaging free radicals. Palm and coconut oils have additional health benefits. They are very rich in lauric acid, which your body converts to monolaurin, which contains antibacterial and antiviral properties. Fats from grass-fed animals contain conjugated linoleic acid (CLA), which is anti-inflammatory and protects against heart disease, and has been shown to lower cancer risk and shrink tumors.

Trans-fats include hydrogenated fats and are part of many processed foods such as commercially made snacks like cookies, doughnuts cakes, crackers, chips, and candy bars. They are also found in commercially fried foods such as fried chicken and chicken nuggets, and French fries and hydrogenated fats like margarine and shortening. Hydrogenated palm and hydrogenated coconut oil fall in this category, turning a good food into a bad one.

Even if it were possible to rid our diets of fat, we shouldn't. Vitamins A, D, E, and K are fat-soluble, meaning they can only be digested, absorbed, and transported in conjunction with fats. Fats are also sources of essential fatty acids, an important dietary requirement.

Omega 3 and Omega 6 are essential fatty acids, or EFAs, that humans and other animals must eat because the body requires them for good health and our bodies cannot manufacture them. The balance between omega-3 and omega-6 fatty acids is very important. The ratio in our diet between these two fatty acids should be somewhere between a 1:1 and a 4:1 omega-6 to omega-3 ratio. Incredibly, average North Americans consume ratios of anywhere from 8:1 to 50:1! We need to decrease omega-6 consumption and increase omega-3 consumption.

Most of us struggle to raise our omega-3 intake to balance out this ratio. So look for omega-6 in the polyunsaturated vegetable oils (safflower, sunflower, corn, sesame, grape-seed, peanut, etc.), mono-unsaturated oils (olive) and avocados, macadamia nuts, almonds, hazelnuts, and pecans. And consciously boost your omega-3 intake (particularly by eating oily fish and fish oils, including cod liver oil, free-range eggs or omega 3 fortified eggs, walnuts, flax seeds, and grass-fed beef.

Personally, I use olive oil for the omega 6 and add 4 grams of fish oil daily to my diet for the omega 3.

FIBER

Fiber refers to carbohydrates that cannot be digested. Fiber is present in all plants that are eaten for food, including fruits, vegetables, grains, and legumes. Fiber decreases risk of heart disease, diabetes, diverticular diseases, and constipation.

Fiber is an important part of a healthy diet, and you should get at least 20 grams a day—but more is better. Most Americans eat less than 15 grams per day. Compared to low fiber foods, foods with fiber help you feel full, so you are less likely to overeat. The best sources are whole grain foods, fresh fruits and vegetables, legumes and nuts.

Both soluble and insoluble fibers are essential to any diet. Examples of soluble fiber include oatmeal, oat-bran, nuts, seeds, legumes, beans, dried peas, lentils, apples, pears, strawberries, and blueberries. Insoluble fibers, which have a laxative effect, include whole wheat bread, barley, couscous, brown rice, bulgur, whole grain breakfast cereals, wheat bran, seeds, carrots, cucumbers, zucchini, celery, and tomatoes.

Here are some tips for increasing your fiber intake:
- Eat whole fruits instead of drinking fruit juices.
- Replace white rice, bread, and pasta with brown rice and whole grain products.
- Choose whole grain cereals for breakfast.
- Snack on raw vegetables instead of chips, crackers, or chocolate bars.
- Substitute legumes for meat two to three times per week in chili and soups.
- Experiment with international dishes (such as Indian or Middle Eastern) that use whole grains and legumes as part of the main meal (as in Indian dahls) or in salads (for example, tabbouleh).

MULTI-VITAMINS AND MINERALS

Even the very best foods grown on earth aren't the same foods that your great-grandparents ate. The abuse of the soils by the big agricultural companies by over-cultivation, the over-use of pesticides and chemical fertilizers, and mineral depletion have led to a soil that is no longer as rich in nutrients as the soil our great-grandparents enjoyed. Not surprisingly, the vegetables and fruits they enjoyed were also much tastier than what we have today. Genetically-modified produce, fewer and fewer types of crops even cultivated, and increased time and distance from the farm to the table decreases the amount of nutrients even available in our foods.

It's important to eat the best foods available to you, but realize that not all your nutritional needs are being met anymore. You should include a high quality multi-vitamin and mineral supplement in your routine for better results in your health, and be sure to make it very high quality because many vitamin manufacturers are using synthetic vitamins to cut costs.

The majority of vitamins that are sold in pharmacies, grocery stores, and vitamin shops are synthetic (man-made) vitamins, which are only isolated portions of the vitamins that occur naturally in food. Synthetic or partial vitamins do not perform the same functions in your body as vitamins found naturally in whole food.

A good example is vitamin C. Real vitamin C found in real food is made up of these components: rutin, bioflavonoids (vitamin P), Factor K, Factor J, Factor P, tyrosinase, ascorbinogen, and ascorbic acid. If you take a look at a variety of vitamin C supplements, you will find that the majority of them contain only ascorbic acid or a compound called ascorbate, which is a less acidic form of ascorbic acid. Ascorbic acid is *not* vitamin C. It is only one part out of eight components that make up real vitamin C. Since vitamins work in conjunction with other vitamins and minerals, the synergy of all the parts working together will be best for your overall health.

So, when choosing a multi-vitamin supplement and mineral supplement, it is in your best interest to use only those products that list actual foods as their ingredients rather than synthetic and isolated vitamins—such as acerola cherry powder instead of just Vitamin C. Get to know your health food store and inquire about the most trusted brands.

BCAA

Branched Chain Amino Acids (BCAAs) are made up of 3 essential amino acids that cannot be produced by your body. BCAAs can make up one-third of skeletal muscle, so they are an important part of your supplement routine.

Taking BCAA supplements will help prevent muscle loss and will encourage visceral fat loss. Visceral fat is that deadly fat that accumulates around your organs in your belly—a definite health hazard! You can maximize your weight loss and retain your muscle mass because supplemental BCAA is rapidly absorbed into the bloodstream.

Since BCAA is especially beneficial in maintaining muscle mass while on a calorie deficit routine, your physique can soon be lean and mean!

Suggested dosage: 5 grams daily.

L-CARNITINE

L-carnitine is a non-essential amino acid—a derivative of the amino acid, lysine—that can be synthesized by the body. Carnitine is a substance that is stored in skeletal muscles where it can be used to transform fatty acids into energy for muscular activity. L-carnitine is often taken to boost exercise performance and studies do show that oral carnitine reduces fat mass, increases muscle mass, and reduces fatigue, which may contribute to weight loss in some people.

Suggested dosage: 2 grams daily.

BETA-ALANINE

Beta-alanine is an amino acid that ups your energy so you can power through your workouts. It can help delay muscle fatigue, promote muscular endurance, and improve workout performance, but only in adequate amounts. Underdoses of 100 mg have absolutely little or no benefit.

Suggested dosage: 3.5 grams daily.

CREATINE

Creatine is an organic acid that is produced naturally in the body from amino acids and transported in the blood for use by our muscles. It is produced primarily in the kidneys and liver and helps to supply energy to all the cells in the body.

Suggested dosage: 3 to 5 grams daily.

PTEROSTILBENE

Pterostilbene is a stilbenoid found in blueberries and grapes. It is a powerful antioxidant that belongs to the group of phytoalexins which are agents produced by plants to fight infections. It is related to resveratrol, a natural phenol whose health benefits of are well known, including anticancer, anti-inflammatory, blood sugar lowering, and other beneficial cardiovascular effects.

Pterostilbene demonstrates a higher bioavailability because it is absorbed into the cell more efficiently. It is thought to have cancer-fighting properties, as well as the ability to fight off and reverse cognitive decline. Studies that used animals fed on blueberry-based diets found significant reduction in blood lipid count and cholesterol count. Pterostilbene was proven in studies to be similar in activity to ciprofibrate, a commercial drug that lowers LDL cholesterol and triglycerides without as many side effects.

Pterostilbene is also believed to have anti-diabetic properties and works as an insulin secretagogue. Insulin secretagogues are simply medicines that work by causing the pancreas to release (or *secrete*) more insulin to help lower your blood sugar.

Suggested dosage: 100 milligrams daily.

LOLA

Two of the best amino acids to add to your daily regimen are L-ornithine and L-aspartate. The ammonia scavenging amino acid salts of L-ornithine assist in fighting fatigue. In a placebo-controlled study using L-ornithine supplementation, subjects using a cycle ergometer were tested for fatigue. The results suggested that L-ornithine has an anti-fatigue effect in increasing the efficiency of energy consumption and promoting the excretion of ammonia, a byproduct of protein metabolism. Unfortunately, all exercise, both anaerobic and aerobic, produces tons of ammonia. And the more ammonia in your blood, the poorer your athletic performance. L-ornithine can help convert ammonia to urea and glutamine and also supports liver function.

L-aspartate is a dicarboxylic amino acid—a protein amino acid naturally found in all life forms. It encourages a healthy metabolism, strengthens the immune system and removes excess toxins from cells. In addition, this type of amino acid helps transport minerals needed to form healthy RNA and DNA to the cells. L-aspartate is also used to treat fatigue and depression, because supplemental aspartate has an anti-fatigue effect on skeletal muscle, Studies have shown that aspartate actually increases stamina and endurance levels in athletes.

Suggested dosage: 1 gram daily.

L-CITRULLINE

L-citrulline is a naturally occurring non-essential amino acid. It aids in protein synthesis for muscle tissue retention and helps to maintain healthy protein balance. Citrulline works along with arginine and ornithine to rid the body of ammonia. L-citrulline can be used alongside arginine to enhance nitric oxide (NO) production. The inner lining of blood vessels use nitric oxide to signal the surrounding smooth muscle to relax. Blood vessels relax and widen and blood flow increases—for a greater workout!

L-citrulline not only promotes lower blood pressure and better circulation—and increases sexual performance—but you also get much fuller muscular pumps when working out as well as a quicker recovery from an intense workout.

Suggested dosage: 3 to 6 grams daily.

ARGININE

Arginine is an amino acid that plays an important role in cell division, the healing of wounds, removing ammonia from the body, immune function, and the release of hormones. It serves many purposes in the body, but one of its most important jobs is to increase nitric oxide in the bloodstream. This causes the blood vessels to relax and increases the flow of blood to the muscles.

Some studies have found that arginine supplements can improve the function of blood vessels, enhance coronary blood flow, lower blood pressure, and even reduce angina and other symptoms in people with heart and/or vascular disease.

Suggested dosage: 6 to 12 grams daily.

ABOUT THE AUTHOR

Rich Gaspari is one of America's foremost professional bodybuilders who was inducted into the International Federation BodyBuilders (IFBB) Hall of Fame in 2004. He is the CEO of Gaspari Nutrition, a sports nutrition company he founded in 2001. His hard-line approach, though novel to industry standards, still stands true—to develop the most useful and effective products in their respective categories while breaking new ground with exciting categories never before seen.

Rich has been featured in numerous fitness and nutrition magazines, including the cover of *Iron Man* (October 2011). His international achievements in bodybuilding are numerous, including winner of the 1989 Arnold Classic and three-time runner-up in the Mr. Olympia competition, recipient of the Arnold Classic Lifetime Achievement Award in 2013 among others. Rich currently lives in New Jersey, where he was born. This is his first book.